Interventional Cardiology in the Elderly

Harald Rittger
Editor

Interventional Cardiology in the Elderly

Springer

Editor
Harald Rittger
Universitatsklinikum Erlangen
Erlangen
Germany

ISBN 978-3-319-21141-1 ISBN 978-3-319-21142-8 (eBook)
DOI 10.1007/978-3-319-21142-8

Library of Congress Control Number: 2015954079

Springer Cham Heidelberg New York Dordrecht London

Printed on acid-free paper

Springer International Publishing AG Switzerland is part of Springer Science+Business Media (www.springer.com)

Contents

Contributors

Philipp Bahrmann Friedrich-Alexander-University, Institute for Biomedicine of Aging, Nürnberg, Germany

Ralf Birkemeyer Interventional Cardiology, Herzklinik Ulm, Ulm, Germany

Thomas Frühwald Geriatric Acute Care Department, Krankenhaus Hietzing mit Neurologischem Zentrum Rosenhügel, Wien, Austria

Christoph Garlichs Medical Clinic, Academic Hospital Flensburg, Flensburg, Germany

Tobias J. Lange Department of Internal Medicine II, University Medical Center Regensburg, Regensburg, Germany

Andreas May Department of Internal Medicine, Klinikum Memmingen, Memmingen, Germany

Harald Rittger Department of Internal Medicine I, Cardiology and Pneumology, Klinikum Fuerth, Fuerth, Germany

Chapter 1
Epidemiology of Coronary Heart Disease in the Elderly

Christoph Garlichs

Introduction

The percentage of people aged 65 years and older in the United States is calculated to increase from 12.4 % (35 million) of the population in 2000 to 19.6 % (71 million) by 2030, with 82 million in that age group by 2050. The number of people older than 80 years of age is projected to double from 9.3 million in 2000 to 19.5 million in 2030, and to more than triple by 2050 [1]. Global trends are similar, with the worldwide population older than 65 years projected to increase to 973 million, or 12 %, in 2030 and to constitute approximately 20 % of the population in 2050 (see also Center of Disease Control [www.cdc.gov] and European Cardiovascular Disease statistic [http://www.ehnheart.org/cvd-statistics.html]). These numbers and dynamics in the development of cardiovascular diseases underscore the necessity for an efficient primary and secondary prevention in the elderly patients.

Atherosclerosis as the driving force of coronary artery disease starts at early ages in life and is universally present in patients above 65 years old. Thereby age is the most important (and uninfluenced) risk factor for the development of atherosclerosis and other heart diseases, so that the demographic shift towards an older population will result in dramatically changed clinical and economic needs in order to provide adequate medical care for this population. For example, the economic costs for the diagnosis and treatment of cardiovascular disease (including stroke) are estimated as high as 315 billions US-Dollar in 2014. The demographic shift will double these cost in 2030 [2].

This chapter about the epidemiology of coronary artery disease in the elderly focuses on the burden of the disease, on subclinical and clinical manifestations, on relevant risk factors for CAD in the elderly, and current available evidences with regard to the management in the primary and secondary prevention of CAD.

C. Garlichs
Medical Clinic, Academic Hospital Flensburg, Flensburg, Germany
e-mail: Christoph.Garlichs@gmx.de

H. Rittger (ed.), *Interventional Cardiology in the Elderly*,
DOI 10.1007/978-3-319-21142-8_1

Clincial Manifestation of Coronary Artery Disease

The lifetime's risk to develop coronary artery disease is quite high. At the age of seventy the risk for a first cardiovascular event is 34.9 % in men and 24.2 % in women. The average age for a myocardial infarction is 64.5 years in men and 70.3 years in women.

Subclinical Coronary Artery Disease

The majority of older patients does not show any clinical symptoms for a clinically relevant CAD. Nevertheless, in many of these patients subclinical CAD can be detected. For example, the Cardiovascular Health Study (CHS) provided evidence of significant carotid artery stenosis >50 % in adults above 65 years and without any known cardiovascular risk factors in 4.3 % of men (age group between 65 and 74 years) increasing to 10.9 % in men over 85 years as well as in 3.4 % and 11.8 % in women, respectively. Left ventricular hypertrophy as another cardiovascular risk factor was detected in 2.1–6.3 % in men and 1.9–5.2 % in women (in the above mentioned age groups) [3].

When combing several cardiovascular characteristics (ECG abnormalities, ABI <0.9, increased Intima-Media-Thickness, echocardiographic abnormalities, angina pectoris or claudication), a retrospective analysis of the Cardiovascular Health Study could discover a prevalence for subclinical cardiovascular diseases of up to 61 %. In correspondence with these findings, Wong et al. took the MESA Trial and found a prevalence for subclinical atherosclerosis (measured as an increased Intima-Media-Thickness, low ABI, or presence of coronary or abdominal aortic calcifications) in 55 % of men at the age between 45 and 54 years 'old' streichen and a prevalence of 100 % in men at the age between 75 and 84 years (in women, prevalence was 32 % as well as 98 % in the above mentioned age groups). In most cases, calcifications of the abdominal aorta gave a hint for the underlying subclinical atherosclerosis. Aortal calcifications appear in equal numbers in men and women, whereas coronary calcifications appear more often in men [4]. The detection of abdominal aortal calcification was a strong predictor for other markers of subclinical atherosclerosis (increased carotid Intima-Media-Thickness, low ABI, coronary calcification).

Atherogenic Risk Factors

The risk for cardiovascular disease rises dramatically with increasing age. In general more than half of all men and one third of all women at the age of 70 years have a 10 % risk to experience a cardiovascular event within the next 10 years. Data of the Framingham Heart Study shows, that the risk for coronary artery disease can step up as much as 5-fold depending on the number of atherogenic risk factors.

Generally speaking, the well-known atherogenic risk factors in young people keep their atherogenity in older patients, although gender differences have to be considered. For example, an increased systolic blood pressure is strongly associated with CAD in young and old people of both ages, whereas an increased diastolic blood pressure is of only marginal significance in older women.

Hypertension

From a global perspective, hypertension is responsible for the death of more than 7 million people per year, thus being the most important of all risk factors. Hypertension among US-citizens is the most frequent cardiovascular risk factor: it appears in 2/3 of all men above 65 years and in about 80 % of women above 75 years. Younger people (<40 years) more often have an isolated diastolic hypertension (i.e. systolic pressure below 140 mmHg, diastolic above 90 mmHg). At the age of 50 years, systolic hypertension becomes more prominent (either as an isolated systolic hypertension or as a combined systolic/diastolic hypertension). In life's sixth decade, isolated systolic arterial hypertension becomes the dominant subtype. At the age between 60–69 years, about 80 % of all people with hypertension demonstrate an isolated systolic arterial hypertension due to an increased stiffness of the great arteries. Additional risk factors such as diabetes mellitus or chronic renal insufficiency, which can also lead to arterial stiffness, can accelerate the rigidity of great arteries thus causing isolated systolic hypertension even in younger ages.

Meanwhile several studies (e.g. the Framingham Heart Study) stress the superiority of an increased pulse pressure and reduced diastolic blood pressure compared to an isolated systolic hypertension with regard to cardiovascular risk stratification in the elderly. After the age of 50 years, systolic blood pressure rises disproportionate to the diastolic blood pressure. After the age of 60 years, diastolic blood pressure drops further resulting in an increase of pulse pressure. Among the ages between 50 and 70 years, there is a positive correlation of the systolic blood pressure and a negative correlation of the diastolic blood pressure with the risk for CAD. This observation underscores the superiority of the pulse pressure in contrast to the systolic hypertension for the prediction of CAD risk.

Age is another important parameter on the hemodynamic system and therefore strongly influences the risk for CAD. This means, that with increasing age there is a gradual transition from diastolic to systolic hypertension and then to pulse pressure as predictors for CAD risk. In addition it could be shown, that the combination of systolic and diastolic blood pressure was superior to the single use of systolic blood pressure in the risk assessment for CAD. In general, the systolic blood pressure is a better predictor for CAD than diastolic blood pressure in people above 50 years. Nevertheless, the risk for CAD can be strongly influenced by a very high systolic or very low diastolic blood pressure. The National Health and Nutrition Examination Survey (NHANES), for example, has demonstrated, that a diastolic blood pressure below 70 mmHg, which appears in about 30 % of untreated people with isolated systolic hypertension, increases the risk for CAD. Factors associated with low diastolic blood pressure were advanced age, female gender as well as diabetes mellitus, but not state of treatment. A recently published sub analysis of the Framingham Heart Study confirmed these results in 791 individuals with a mean age of 75 years: here, persons with isolated systolic hypertension (and prior CVD events) have increased risk for recurrent CVD events in the presence of diastolic blood pressure <70 mmHg versus DBP 70–89 mmHg, whether treated or untreated, supporting wide pulse pressure as an important risk modifier for the adverse effect of low diastolic blood pressure [5].

Dyslipidemia

Initial sub analysis of the Framingham Heart Study suggested that no positive correlation exists between serum cholesterol levels and CAD risk in older men. Meanwhile, some studies could prove, that serum cholesterol levels strongly predict new as well as recurrent cardiovascular events in older men and women. For example, Aronow et al. proved in a study with a 40–48 months follow-up with groups of 644 older men and 1488 older women a 12 % increase in the risk for cardiovascular events with each 10 mg/dL rise of total cholesterol [6]. In a meta analysis by Manolio et al., based on 22 US and international cohort studies, serum cholesterol levels showed a rather weak predictive power in older men and women. In these studies, the frailty and comorbidity of patients strongly influenced the results, so after adjusting for these factors, total cholesterol regained predictive power for future cardiovascular events [7].

With regard to HDL cholesterol, Castelli et al showed an inverse correlation between low HDL cholesterol and new coronary events [8]. A similar association was shown in the above mentioned study by Aronow et al., in which a 70 % increased risk for cardiovascular events in men and a 95 % increased risk in women was seen with every descent of 10 mg/dL of HLD cholesterol. Additional results of this study showed, that hypertriglyceridemia is only a weak risk factor in women, but not in men. Whereas total cholesterol did not consistently prove to be a predictor for CAD events, the determination of HDL cholesterol or the relation between total cholesterol/HDL cholesterol consistently proved to be an important predictor for CAD risk.

What about the potential benefits of pharmacological interventions in elderly patients with hypercholesterolemia? Several studies could show that the effectiveness of such lipid lowering interventions is comparable to those in younger patients. For example, in the well-known 4S Study (Scandinavian Simvastatin Survival Study), a placebo-controlled study in high risk patients (the majority of which had proven CAD), the treatment with a statin (simvastatin) lead to a 43 % reduction of CAD mortality in subjects above 65 years as compared to subjects below 65 years. Moreover, the CARE-Study (Cholesterol and Recurrent Events Study) proved, that a statin therapy was even more effective in patients above 65 years in reducing cardiovascular events (32 % risk reduction) in comparison to the risk reduction in patients below 65 years (19 % risk reduction).

Altogether, there are only a few studies about lipid interventions specifically in older patients. One of these studies is the PROSPER-study performed in men and women between the age of 70–82 years and a history or risk factors for vascular diseases. These patients were treated with the statin 'Pravastatin' (40 mg/day; n=2.891) or placebo (n=2.913). After an average follow-up of 3.2 years the primary end point was analysed (i.e. a combined end point of coronary death, non-fatal myocardial infarction and fatal or non-fatal stroke). Pravastatin reduced LDL-cholesterol by 34 % and thereby significantly reduced the incidence of the primary endpoint (hazard ration 0.85, 95 % CI, 0.74–0.97, p=0.014). It also reduced coronary death and the risk for non-fatal myocardial infarctions (0.81, 0.69–0. 94, p=0.006). Surprisingly, new cancer disease appeared significantly more often in patients treated with pravastatin as compared to the placebo group (1.25, 1.04–1.51, p=0.02). In the meantime, several metaanalyses of studies using pravastatin or other statins could convincingly eliminate any increased incidence of risk for cancer under chronic statin therapy. At last, the Cholesterol Treatment Trialist' Collaboration with more than 170,000 patients in 26 studies has to be mentioned. This trial showed a 22 % general benefit of a lipid lowering therapy for the reduction in CAD events. No significant differences were seen in the age group below 65 years, 65–74 years, and older than 75 years. In addition, this study shows a rather weak effect of a lipid lowering therapy in very old patients (i.e. only a 16 % risk reduction).

Metabolic Syndrome and Diabetes

According to the American Heart Association/National Heart, Lung, and Blood Institute (NHLBI), the diagnosis of a metabolic syndrome is made in the presence of three or more of the following factors: (A) abdominal adiposity defined as a hip size above 102 cm in men and above 88 cm in women, (B) elevated blood pressure (>130 mmHg systolic or >85 mmHg diastolic or treated with antihypertensive drugs), (C) fasting blood glucose of 100 mg/dL and more or treated with antihyperglycemic agents, (D) HDL-cholesterol below 40 mg/dL in men or below 50 mg/dL in women or ongoing treatment due to a low HDL-cholesterol, and (E) fasting triglycerides of 150 mg/dL or higher or ongoing triglyceride-lowering treatment [9].

The prevalence of the metabolic syndrome in adults drastically increases with age (about 50 % of men at the age of 65 suffer from it). The prevalence in diabetes, defined as a fasting glucose of 126 mg/dL or above or ongoing antihyperglycaemic therapy, rises with age as well, with a rate of about 20 % in patients in the age of 65 years. The life-time risk for diabetes is estimated between 25 and 45 % in women and 30–55 % in men, whereby ethnical difference exert a strong influence (in the US, for example, US-Americans Hispanics develop far more often diabetes as compared to non-Hispanic whites). In analogy with the observation, that cardiovascular risk factors increase with age, do people with metabolic syndrome or diabetes mellitus have a 20 % elevated 10-years risk for the development of coronary artery disease or cardiovascular disease in general. And about 80 % of people with diabetes at the age above 60 years have a 20 % cardiovascular risk or already a diagnosed cardiovascular disease.

Without any doubts, diabetes is an important risk factor for coronary events in older men and women and associated with a 2-fold risk for new coronary events according to a study based on 644 older men and 1488 older women (i.e. a study with a follow-up of 40–48 months). In addition, the Framingham Heart Study demonstrated that an elevated fasting glucose and the composite endpoint of glucose intolerance and diabetes are a strong risk factor for new coronary events in an observation period of 30 years.

Up to now, there has been no larger study demonstrating the benefit of an intensive blood glucose control in older patients with diabetes on future cardiovascular events. But there a subanalyses of larger studies, which help to clarify the potential clinical benefit of an intensive blood glucose control in these patients. The ADVANCE-Study, for example, consisted of 11,140 persons with diabetes mellitus type 2 and a median follow-up of 5.0 years, and an intensive control of blood glucose with a target of a HbA1c below 6.5 % led to a 30 % reduction of larger microvascular and macrovascular events. This benefit was seen in people below and above the age of 65 years (although no statistical significance was reached in the latter and no risk reduction for major macrovascular events was seen in the whole study) [10]. The later results are in accordance with the ACCORD-Study (The Action to Control Cardiovascular Risk in Diabetes), where no benefit of an intensive blood glucose control was seen in 10,251 younger and older persons, which either received standard or an intensified therapy (with a target value of HbA1c <6 %) [11]. Noteworthy is the fact that patients with new onset diabetes mellitus or no signs of macrovascular disease at study entrance showed the greatest benefit of a treatment.

Thus individualization of therapy becomes important. For selected individual patients, lower HbA1c goals than the general goal of <7.0 % should be considered if this can be achieved without significant hypoglycaemia or other adverse effects of treatment (i.e. in patients with short duration of diabetes, long life expectancy, and no significant cardiovascular disease). Conversely, less stringent HbA1c goals than the general goal <7 % may be appropriate for patients with a history of severe hypoglycaemia, limited life expectancy, advanced microvascular or macrovascular cardiovascular disease, extensive comorbid conditions, or those with long-standing diabetes. Since there is a high prevalence of these characteristics in the elderly patients, the later approach should to be favoured [12].

Smoking

Initial analysis of the Framingham Heart Study did not show any association of cigarette smoking with coronary artery disease in patients above the age of 60. By contrast, the Honolulu Heart Study proved a 2-fold increase risk for CAD in male cigarette smokers at the age of 65–74 years and in 644 male and 1488 female people with a mean age of 80 years (40–48 months follow up) [13].

With regard to secondary prevention, studies (for example the Coronary Artery Surgery Study, CASS study) showed a 1.5-fold increased risk for myocardial infarction and death in patients at the age between 65 and 69 years. This risk even increased to 2.9 in patients above 70 years as well as in persistent smokers compared to former smokers. Moreover, the CASS study demonstrated an increased 6-years-mortality rate (relative risk about 1.7) in persons with persistent nicotine abuse in comparison to former smokers, who had to quit at least 1 year before study entrance [14]. Interestingly, the benefit of quitting smoking was detectable in all age groups. In summary these studies underscore that resigning from smoking reduces the risk of myocardial infarction und increases life expectancy in younger as well as in older people.

Overweight and Adiposity

A few studies identified adiposity as a risk factor for secondary coronary events in elderly patients with coronary artery disease. Former prospective studies had already shown, that obesity in general and central obesity in particular is a risk factor for the incidence of CAD in men and women in the mean age. But there are only a few studies available about the influence of obesity in elderly patients. Data from the Framingham Heart Study suggest that CAD in elderly patients is associated with similar atherogenic risk factors as seen in younger patients. Nevertheless some specific characteristics seem to exist in the elderly: the Honolulu Heart Program as well as the Health Professionals Follow-Up Study (HPFS) have shown that weight gain in adults below 65 years has a stronger positive correlation with risk for CAD as compared to weight gain in men above 65 years. This finding can partially be explained by the well described substitution of muscle with fat tissue in elderly people. In addition, this phenomenon may account for the observation of previous cohort studies in elderly people, in which only moderate or no correlations were seen between body mass index and CAD risk. The latter studies also identified hip size and fat distribution as strong predictors for cardiovascular events. In one of these studies, Rimm's analysis of the HPFS data observed that in men above 65 years only a weak correlation existed between body mass index and CAD risk, whereas a strong correlation existed between waist-to-hip ratio and CAD risk (relative risk 2.7) [15]. This was due to the increased mass of abdominal fat with increasing age, revealing the body mass index as a bad indicator for the general fat mass in elderly patients. Moreover, corresponding randomized studies proved that lifestyle interventions by diet-induced weight reduction and physical training leads to an improvement of obesity-associated CAD risk factors in overweight elderly patients [16]. Altogether, this data from several studies shows that CAD risk factors (such as hip size, hypertension, circulating inflammatory substances, pathological glucose tolerance, insulin resistance, fasting glucose levels, and lipids) are reversible not only in younger patients, but also in elderly, overweight patients.

Physical Activity

Reduced physical fitness and physical activity is predictive for a higher mortality rate in older persons. These observations are independent of obesity and abdominal adiposity and have resulted in recommendations for frequent physical activity in older adults. In addition, physical activity is a significant predictor for the risk of CAD. Data from the Honolulu Heart Program showed a 2.2 fold increased risk for cardiovascular events in people who walked less than 500 m/day as compared to people with a daily course of 2 km. Similar results were obtained in the Harvard Alumni Study, in which men at the age of 66 years, who consumed about 4000 kcal/week through physical activity (walking, sports, stair climbing), had a 38 % reduced relative risk for CAD when compared to men who consumed less than 1000 kcal/week. This study also demonstrated that the duration of the physical activity did not influence the relative risk as far as the amount of consumed energy was equal.

Frequent physical activity has been favourable for the general cardiovascular health in elderly patients. Data about 1645 men and women at the age above 65 years documents, that – after adjusting for cardiovascular risk factors – walking for more than 4 h/week results in a significant reduced risk for cardiovascular-caused hospitalization (relative risk of 0.69) as compared to walking of less than 1 h/week. It has to be mentioned that these studies included only a small fraction of people above the age of 80 years. Nevertheless, these studies show, that physical exercise in elderly people has a beneficial effect on CAD risk similar to that in younger adults.

Physical activity in the context of secondary prevention has been proved to be effective in the reduction of CAD-caused mortality. The British Regional Heart Study observed that the lowest risk for cardiovascular mortality was seen in CAD patients with slight to moderate physical activity (relative risk of 0.42 and 0.47, respectively) as compared to physical inactive people or people with only occasional physical activity. Thereby, physical activity in the form of regular walking or intense gardening seemed to more effective than sport activities [17].

Inflammatory Risk Factors

The concentration of inflammatory markers increases with age; this is mainly due to a decrease in sexual hormones and an increase in visceral fat. Whether inflammatory markers have to be considered as independent risk factors for coronary artery disease is currently still a matter of debate. Thereby, many studies have established C-reactive protein as an acute inflammatory marker that plays a significant role in cardiovascular diseases. In 2002, the American Heart Association recommend CRP as a useful screening marker for patients with an intermediate risk for cardiovascular events within the next 10 years [18].

Preventive Strategies

Primary Prevention

Prevention of CAD in elderly patients involves not only primary and secondary prevention, but also primordial preventive strategies with the aim to avoid the development of the atherogenic risk factors. This explains the program by the American Heart Association, in which 'seven easy goals' focus on the preservation of normal lipid values, blood glucose levels, body fat, and the avoidance of smoking and taking of a healthy diet and regular physical activity. In this context, data of the NHANES from 2007 to 2008 is interesting, which shows that elderly patients fewest reached the above mentioned 'seven easy goals'; patients above 60 years had the lowest percentage of all age classes with regard to obtaining at least 4 or more of the mentioned criteria; and only 10 % fulfilled 4 criteria and only 5 % 5–6 criteria of altogether 7 possible goals.

Adequate blood pressure control as well as lipid control proved to have a beneficial effect in all age classes. Since elderly patients possess a particular high risk for cardiovascular events, therapeutic interventions to control atherogenic risk factors seem to be at least as important as in younger adults. Interventions to control atherogenic risk factors in the elderly induce a dramatic reduction of the absolute risk for CAD. According to a study by Wong et al., optimal management of blood lipids and blood pressure in adults with metabolic syndrome resulted in an 80 % reduction of coronary events (an effect, which was seen in all age groups) [19]. Thereby therapy of high blood pressure as the most important risk factor for mortality worldwide is of particular importance in the elderly.

Risk factor control has to include life style modifications such as reduction of daily intake of sodium, adjusting body weight, an only moderate consumption of alcohol as well as regular physical activity, all of which being factors easing the control of elevated blood pressure. In addition, studies proved the benefit of quitting to smoke even in elderly patients.

Secondary Prevention

Secondary prevention of chronic heart disease in the elderly naturally embraces the discussed risk factors relevant for primary prevention. However, relatively few studies have been reported about the effectiveness of theses interventions in older patients.

Smoking cessation leads to numerous benefits in patients with cardiovascular disease. Most of all, it reduces overall mortality by 25–50 % in those who have suffered an myocardial infarction, and at least 50 % of this decline is seen in the first year. In older patients who have undergone CABG surgery, smoking cessation reduced both morbidity and mortality rates (data from CASS study). Since smoking cessation rate (in middle-aged and older persons) range from 20 to 70 % after 1 year, conclusive multiple components programs are needed to convince patients about the benefits of smoking cessation.

With regard to antihypertensive therapy, metaanalyses have demonstrated the particularly high benefits in patients 60–80 years in age. Antihypertensive treatment prevents strokes and heart failure more than coronary events, but overall mortality also is reduced. The general target should be <140/90 mmHg. For patients with heart failure, renal insufficiency and diabetes, a lower target such as <130 mmHg is recommended.

Strategies for lipid-lowering therapy in the elderly can be derived from several subanalyses of Statin trials. The 4S-trial showed similar reductions in CHD mortality and hospitalization in patients >65 years of age compared with younger patients. The CARE Study demonstrated that statin therapy was equally effective in older patients with known CHD and a total cholesterol <240 mg/dL (32 % risk reduction compared with 19 % risk reduction). For CHD deaths, the difference was even more striking (reduction in CHD mortality 11 % in patients <65 years versus 45 % in patients >65 years). Because mortality rates increase substantially with age, the elderly derived a greater absolute benefit (for every 1000 patients treated, 225 cardiovascular hospitalizations would be prevented compared with 121 hospitalizations in 1000 younger patients).

Obesity is another starting point for secondary prevention in the elderly according to the Framingham study. This is primarily due to the prominent clustering of dyslipidaemia, hypertension, and insulin resistance in older overweight individuals and particularly in individuals with preferential abdominal obesity. Therefore, weight reduction can result in a multifactorial risk reduction intervention in obese patients.

Several studies have shown that exercise training alone without a nutritional approach has only a minimal effect on measures of obesity and abdominal adiposity in older coronary patients [20]. This is probably due to the low exercise-related energy expenditure accomplished by patients with CHD in general and particularly by older patients. Altogether there are only a few studies among the elderly with CHD which provide convincing data about the effect of weight reduction on secondary cardiovascular events. In one of these studies in obese patients with a mean age of 60 with CHD, hypocaloric diet-induced weight reduction of 11 kg resulted in a 10 % lowering in total and LDL-cholesterol, 24 % lowering of triglycerides, and an 8 % gain in HDL-cholesterol [21].

Diabetes is another strong predictor for secondary cardiovascular events in older CHD patients. Despite the lack of data with regard to the efficacy of treating diabetes in the elderly the management of diabetes seems to be important in this subgroup in order to prevent micro- and macrovascular complications. Appropriate medical therapy to achieve near-normal fasting plasma glucose with an official goal of HbA1c <7 % is recommended.

Conclusions

The main burden of costs for hospitalisation due to coronary artery disease is caused by people above the age of 65. The above mentioned lives modifications allow prevention and reduction in the development of atherogenic risk factors such as arterial hypertension, dyslipidaemia, and diabetes mellitus. In addition, pharmacological therapy can adequately treat hypertension and the other atherogenic risk factors. Studies have sufficiently proved that life modification and pharmacological treatment are also effective in elderly patients. With this means we can treat elderly patients resulting in healthier lives and longer periods without cardiovascular events. These means have proven to be effective in elderly patients even in secondary prevention. It depends on us, whether or not we will apply our current knowledge on preventive measures in order to improve the quality of life as well as life expectancy of elderly patients.

References

1. Douglas L, Mann DPZ, Peter L, Bonow RO. Braunwald's Heart disease. A Textbook of cardiovascular medicine. Braunwald's Heart disease. 10th ed. Verlag: Saunders W.B.; Auflage: 10th edition. 2014. Expert Consult - Online and Print. (18. September 2014).
2. Go AS, Mozaffarian D, Roger VL, Benjamin EJ, Berry JD, Blaha MJ, et al. Heart disease and stroke statistics – 2014 update: a report from the American Heart Association. Circulation. 2014;129:e28–292.
3. Bild DE, Fitzpatrick A, Fried LP, Wong ND, Haan MN, Lyles M, et al. Age-related trends in cardiovascular morbidity and physical functioning in the elderly: the Cardiovascular Health Study. J Am Geriatr Soc. 1993;41:1047–56.
4. Wong ND, Lopez VA, Allison M, Detrano RC, Blumenthal RS, Folsom AR, et al. Abdominal aortic calcium and multi-site atherosclerosis: the Multiethnic Study of Atherosclerosis. Atherosclerosis. 2011;214:436–41.
5. Franklin SS, Gokhale SS, Chow VH, Larson MG, Levy D, Vasan RS, et al. Does low diastolic blood pressure contribute to the risk of recurrent hypertensive cardiovascular disease events?: the Framingham Heart Study. Hypertension. 2015;65:299–305.
6. Aronow WS, Ahn C. Risk factors for new coronary events in a large cohort of very elderly patients with and without coronary artery disease. Am J Cardiol. 1996;77:864–6.
7. Manolio TA, Pearson TA, Wenger NK, Barrett-Connor E, Payne GH, Harlan WR. Cholesterol and heart disease in older persons and women. Review of an NHLBI workshop. Ann Epidemiol. 1992;2:161–76.
8. Castelli WP, Wilson PW, Levy D, Anderson K. Cardiovascular risk factors in the elderly. Am J Cardiol. 1989;63:12H–9.
9. Grundy SM. Metabolic syndrome scientific statement by the American Heart Association and the National Heart, Lung, and Blood Institute. Arterioscler Thromb Vasc Biol. 2005;25:2243–4.
10. Group AC, Patel A, MacMahon S, Chalmers J, Neal B, Billot L, et al. Intensive blood glucose control and vascular outcomes in patients with type 2 diabetes. N Engl J Med. 2008; 358:2560–72.
11. Action to Control Cardiovascular Risk in Diabetes Study G, Gerstein HC, Miller ME, Byington RP, Goff Jr DC, Bigger JT, et al. Effects of intensive glucose lowering in type 2 diabetes. N Engl J Med. 2008;358:2545–59.
12. Giorgino F, Leonardini A, Laviola L. Cardiovascular disease and glycemic control in type 2 diabetes: now that the dust is settling from large clinical trials. Ann N Y Acad Sci. 2013; 1281:36–50.
13. Benfante R, Reed D, Frank J. Does cigarette smoking have an independent effect on coronary heart disease incidence in the elderly? Am J Public Health. 1991;81:897–9.
14. Hermanson B, Omenn GS, Kronmal RA, Gersh BJ. Beneficial six-year outcome of smoking cessation in older men and women with coronary artery disease. Results from the CASS registry. N Engl J Med. 1988;319:1365–9.

15. Rimm EB, Stampfer MJ, Giovannucci E, Ascherio A, Spiegelman D, Colditz GA, et al. Body size and fat distribution as predictors of coronary heart disease among middle-aged and older US men. Am J Epidemiol. 1995;141:1117–27.
16. Villareal DT, Miller 3rd BV, Banks M, Fontana L, Sinacore DR, Klein S. Effect of lifestyle intervention on metabolic coronary heart disease risk factors in obese older adults. Am J Clin Nutr. 2006;84:1317–23.
17. Wannamethee SG, Shaper AG, Walker M. Physical activity and mortality in older men with diagnosed coronary heart disease. Circulation. 2000;102:1358–63.
18. Pearson TA. AHA guidelines for primary prevention of cardiovascular disease and stroke: 2002 update: consensus panel guide to comprehensive risk reduction for adult patients without coronary or other atherosclerotic vascular diseases. Circulation. 2002;106:388–91.
19. Wong ND, Pio JR, Franklin SS, L'Italien GJ, Kamath TV, Williams GR. Preventing coronary events by optimal control of blood pressure and lipids in patients with the metabolic syndrome. Am J Cardiol. 2003;91:1421–6.
20. Lavie CJ, Milani RV. Effects of cardiac rehabilitation and exercise training on exercise capacity, coronary risk factors, behavioral characteristics, and quality of life in women. Am J Cardiol. 1995;75:340–3.
21. Katzel LI, Coon PJ, Dengel J, Goldberg AP. Effects of an American Heart Association step I diet and weight loss on lipoprotein lipid levels in obese men with silent myocardial ischemia and reduced high-density lipoprotein cholesterol. Metabolism. 1995;44:307–14.

Chapter 2
Pathophysiology of the Aging Heart and Its Impact on Interventions

Harald Rittger

This chapter will briefly explain, why an understanding of the physiological changes in an elderly cardiovascular system is essential to understand age-dependant alterations in coronary pathology. Especially in the presence of atherosclerosis and its resulting impact on coronary and structural interventions. According to Cheitlin et al. [1], these physiological changes in cardiovascular physiology have to be differentiated from the effects of pathology, such as coronary artery disease, that frequently results with increasing age. These age related changes occur in everyone, however not necessarily at the same rate, consequently leading to variations seen in some people between chronological age and physiological age [1].

Age related changes to the cardiovascular system are summarized in the table (Table 2.1):

Physiological aging is a complex process resulting in severe changes to cardiovascular structures. To begin with, there are alterations to the heart muscle itself: developing into a hypertrophic muscle that is less responsive to sympathetic stimulation, however not to parasympathetic stimulation. The hypertrophy is caused by increasing fibrosis, dropout and apoptosis of myocytes and subsequently leading to a decrease in left ventricular compliance resulting in diastolic dysfunction. Therefore additional mechanisms are necessary to maintain cardiac output, for instance the additional use of the Frank-Starling mechanism or the increased utilization of the atrial contraction for left ventricular filling. This phenomenon appears to be the primary factor for the development of heart failure with a maintained ejection fraction in the elderly. Especially in specific situations such as a new onset of atrial fibrillation or fluid overload, as in long lasting PCI-maneuvers.

The second major issue is the decreasing elasticity of the major arteries, which makes the aorta and the big arteries elongated and stiffer. Subsequently enhancing

H. Rittger, MD
Department of Internal Medicine I, Cardiology and Pneumology, Klinikum Fuerth, Fuerth, Germany
e-mail: harald.rittger@uk-erlangen.de

H. Rittger (ed.), *Interventional Cardiology in the Elderly*,
DOI 10.1007/978-3-319-21142-8_2

Table 2.1 Effects of aging on major structural and functional characteristics of the cardiovascular system

Cardiac changes		Vascular changes	
Heart weight	↑	Arterial wall thickness (intima-media)	↑
Cardiomyocyte dimensions	↑	Subendothelial collagen	↑
Cardiomyocyte number	↓	Elastin	↑
Collagen in cross-linking	↑	Elastin fragmentation	↑
Ejection fraction	=	Proteoglycans	↑
Stroke volume	=	MMP activity	↑
Cardiac output	=	Intimai migration/proliferation of VSMC	↑
Early diastolic filling	↓	Arterial distensibility	↓
End-diastolic filling	↑	Pulse wave velocity	↑
Chronotropic responsiveness to β-adrenergic stimuli/catecholamines	↓	Total peripheral resistance	↑
Inotropic responsiveness to β-adrenergic stimuli/catecholamines	↓	Endothelial permeability	↑
Inotropic response to digitalis glycosides	↓	Endothelial nitric oxide release	↓
Peak cardiac output to maximal effort	↓	Inflammatory markers/mediators	↑
Lusitropic function	↓	SOD activity	↓
Release of natriuretic peptides	↑	β-Adrenergic-mediated vasodilation	↓

Adapted from Ferrrari et al. with permission. (see Ref. [2])
↓ diminished, ↑ augmented, = unchanged, *VSMC* vascular smooth muscle cells, *SOD* superoxide dismutase, *MMP* matrix metallo-proteinases

the pulse wave velocity which leads to increased antegrade and retrograde pulse wave reflections. As a result blood pressure the diastolic blood pressure is noticeable. These phenomenons coincide with endothelial dysfunction and abnormal biochemical patterns causing early atherosclerosis. As a result, vessels are more twisted and calcified with an increased risk of dissection and perforation. However, not only access-site- or coronary vessels are affected. Vessel changes also affect main vessels such as the aorta, the cerebrovascular vessels, as well as the renal vessels. Consequently, the elderly are prone to a higher risk of cerebrovascular events and renal failure after catheterization caused by cerebral embolism from calcium and cholesterol plaques, mobilized with catheters and other devices during the access via the aorta.

Furthermore, age related changes in neural cardiovascular control are likely to be responsible for inadequate baroreceptor and blood pressure responses, potentially resulting in an increased blood pressure variability with accompanying reduced heart rate variability.

Responsiveness to ß-adrenergic stimulation is diminished and both catecholamine- or exercise induced increases in heart rate and myocardial contractility are decreased in elderly patients. Subsequently, as already mentioned, the elderly mechanism needs additional contractile reserves to establish a stable cardiac output.

In a paper Julius et al. state, that the aging heart performs like a younger heart on ß-blocker treatment [3].

In addition to that, fibrosis and calcification of the fibrous heart skeleton lead to calcification of the annular rings and aortic cusps as well as the leaflets of the mitral valves. A dropout of the atrial pacemaker cells result in a decrease in the intrinsic heart rate. With fibrosis of the cardiac skeleton, there is also calcification at the base of the aortic valve and thus damage to the His bundle as it perforates the right fibrous trigone. Finally there is a decreased responsiveness to beta adrenergic receptor stimulation, a decreased reactivity to baroreceptors and chemoreceptors, and an increase in circulating catecholamines [4]. According to Cheitlin et al., these changes set the stage for isolated systolic hypertension, diastolic dysfunction and heart failure, atrioventricular conduction defects and aortic valve calcification – all diseases seen in the elderly [1].

In addition to the changes in heart and vessels described briefly in this chapter, changes in other physiological systems like renal function or hemostasis and of course, problems caused by multimedication, have to be taken into account when referring elderly patients to coronary or structural interventions. In this context, the changes in renal function are of special interest. Creatinin clearance declines by about 50 % between the third and the ninth decade, albeit causing minimal changes in serum creatinin levels. This decline in creatinin clearance is caused by the following: a loss of renal parenchyma, a reduction in renal plasma flow and a reduction in renal hormone activity such as plasma renin and plasma aldosterone.

All these changes are a result of an aging organism and as stated before this varies greatly from human to human, subsequently resulting in individual differences between the chronological and the biological age. In combination with atherosclerosis all the before mentioned age-dependent changes increase the risk of complications during and after PCI. Moreover, comorbidity and consequently multimedication (due to hyper- or hypothyroidism, diabetes, hypertension and heart failure) can not in all instances be differentiated to be either disease- or age-related. Probably resulting in a less likely impact on the immediate PCI outcome, however with a greater influence on the long term effects desired by elderly patients – not so much to prolong life – but an improvement in functional status, quality of life and activities of daily life.

References

1. Cheitlin MD. Cardiovascular physiology-changes with aging. Am J Geriatr Cardiol. 2003;12:9–13.
2. Ferrari AU, Radaelli A, Centola M. Aging and the cardiovascular system. J Appl Physiol. 2003;95:2591–7.
3. Julius S, Antoon A, Witlock LS, Conway J. Influence of age on the hemodynamic response to exercise. Circulation. 1976;36:222–30.
4. Lean M, Goldber PB, Roberts J. An ultrastructural study of the effects of aging on sympathetic innervation and atrial tissue in the rat. J Mol Cell Cardiol. 1983;15:75–92.

Chapter 3
The Role of Geriatric Preconditions (Frailty and Disability) in Elderly Patients and Its Possible Impact on Interventions

Harald Rittger

Introduction

"Frailty is a syndrome that reflects a state of decreased physiological reserve and vulnerability to stressors" [1]. This statement delineates very accurately the process interventional cardiologists and cardiac surgeons in many cases have to deal with, when treating elderly patients. Frailty is a product of an aging organism, of the environment and additional diseases. With an increasing proportion of patients above 80 years needing treatment for coronary artery disease, a growing percentage of those patients will receive this treatment in the presence of frailty, comorbidity and disability. In a frail organism decreasing organ function and muscular decline lead to a catabolic situation. Figure 3.1 shows two pathways leading to the phenotype of frailty.

Afilalo et al. wrote in a meta-analysis, that frailty is associated with a two- to threefold increase in the prevalence of coronary artery disease (CAD) and is a powerful predictor of mortality in cardiovascular patients independent of age, underlying disease severity, comorbid conditions and disability [1]. In a recent review article the frequency of frailty was reported to be in a range from 10 to 60 %, depending on CVD (cardiovascular disease) burden and definition of frailty [2]. According to Afilalo, "epidemiological studies have consistently demonstrated that frailty carries a relative risk of >2 for mortality and morbidity across a spectrum of stable CVD, acute coronary syndromes, heart failure, surgical and transcatheter interventions" [1] and in patients with CVD frailty causes a two fold increase in mortality [3] Figs. 3.2 and 3.3.

H. Rittger, MD
Department of Internal Medicine I, Cardiology and Pneumology, Klinikum Fuerth, Fuerth, Germany
e-mail: harald.rittger@uk-erlangen.de

H. Rittger (ed.), *Interventional Cardiology in the Elderly*,
DOI 10.1007/978-3-319-21142-8_3

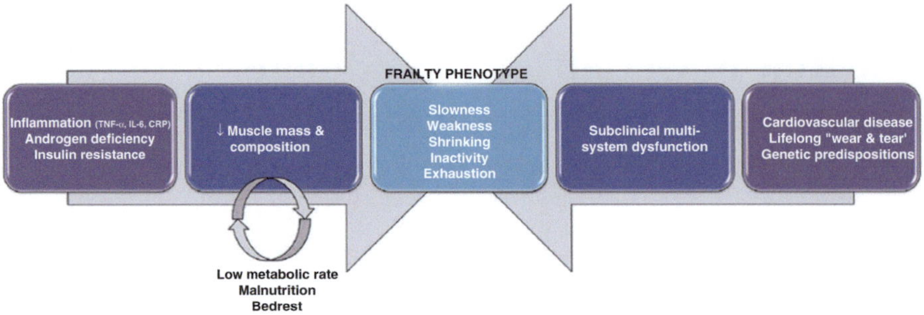

Fig. 3.1 Two pathways leading toward the phenotype of frailty (Adapted from Ref. [1] with permission)

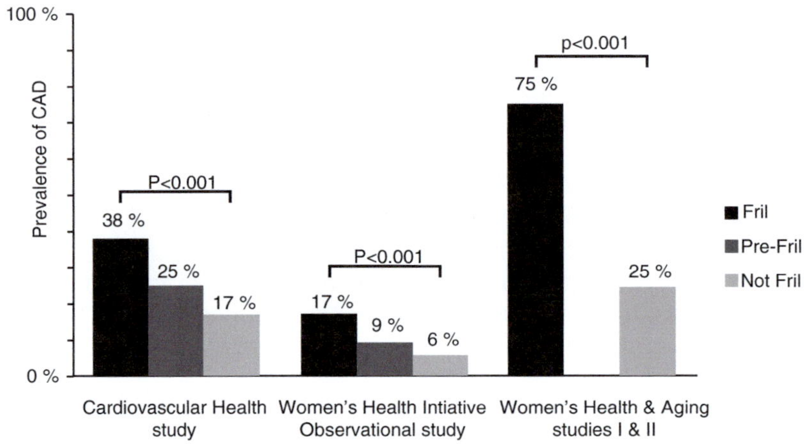

Fig. 3.2 Prevalence of cardiovascular disease stratified by frailty status according to the Fried's criteria (Adapted from Afilalo et al. [1] with permission)

The questions and challenges for interventional cardiologists, treating such patients are:

1. To which extent will the above mentioned preconditions impact the chosen treatment route for cardiac disease (either medical, interventional or surgical).
2. If so, then risk assessment for those patients, who are forwarded to PCI appears crucial in order to identify patients at risk and to re-evaluate treatment strategy.
3. Third and most important, what effect does either therapy or withholding of therapy have in those patients. Does the patient benefit from an intervention or do we cause harm – this question remains unsolved.

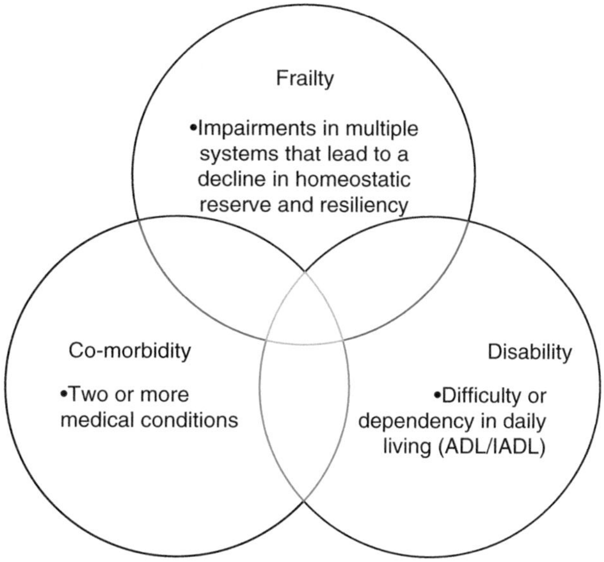

Fig. 3.3 Overlap between frailty, comorbidity and disability. *ADL* activities of daily living, *IADL* instrumental ADL (Adapted from Ref. [1] with permission)

Definition and Measurement

According to Morley JE [4], frailty is a syndrome in which a patient has subclinical impairment of routine activities that exceeds normal age related deterioration. Different measurements of frailty were proposed (Tables 3.1 and 3.2). Fried et al. defined frailty having more than three of the following parameters: weight loss, exhaustion, low activity and slowed walking speed [5].

Up to 20 frailty assessment tools have been developed, with most tools revolving around the core phenotypic domains of frailty: slow walking speed, weakness, inactivity, exhaustion and shrinking – measured by physical performance tests and questionnaires.

Among all these tests, the Fried Scale is predominantly used and best evaluated, including parameters such as slowness, weakness, low physical activity, exhaustion and shrinking (unintentional weight loss) (Ref. [5]).

Another commonly used test is the short physical performance battery (SPPB) [8]. Contrary to the other frailty scales, 5 m gait speed and handgrip strength has been advocated as a single-item measurement of frailty. Especially gait speed seems to have excellent interrater variability [9].

Is it frailty alone, which has to be incorporated into the risk evaluation of patients undergoing coronary intervention or other alternative parameters like gait speed, the "timed-up-and-go-Test" and other specifications like nutritional status, cognition and poor functional status? The extent to which these parameters impact the results, is still under research and consequently needs further evaluation.

Table 3.1 Components of the Fried frailty scale

Shrinking (weight loss)	Shrinking was defined through self-report as an unintentional weight loss of ≥10 pounds in the last year
Decreased grip strength (weakness)	Weakness was assessed by grip strength, and was measured directly with a hand-held JAMAR dynamometer (Sammons Preston Rolyan). Three serial tests of maximum grip strength with the dominant hand were performed, and a mean of the 3 values were adjusted by gender and body mass index (BMI).8,9 Weakness was defined as an adjusted grip strength in the lowest 20th percentile of a community-dwelling population of adults 65 years of age and older. Men met the criteria for weakness if their BMI and grip strength were ≤24 and ≤29 kg; 24.1–26 and ≤30 kg; 26.1–28 and ≤31 kg; >28 and ≤32 kg, respectively. Women met the criteria for weakness if their BMI and grip strength were ≤23 and ≤17 kg; 23.1–26 and ≤17.3 kg; 26.1–29 and ≤18 kg; and >29 and ≤21 kg, respectively
Exhaustion	Exhaustion was measured by responses to the following 2 statements from the modified 10-item Center for Epidemiological Studies–Depression scale [13]: "I felt that everything I did was an effort" and "I could not get going." Subjects were asked, "How often in the last week did you feel this way?" Potential responses were: 0 = rarely or none of the time (<1 day); 1 = some or a little of the time (1–2 days); 2 = a moderate amount of the time (3–4 days); and 3 = most of the time. Subjects answering either statement with response 2 or 3 met the criteria for exhaustion
Low activity	Physical activities were ascertained for the 2 weeks before this assessment using the short version of the Minnesota Leisure Time Activities Questionnaire, and included frequency and duration. Weekly tasks were converted to equivalent kilocalories of expenditure, and individuals reporting a weekly kilocalorie expenditure in the lowest 20th percentile for their gender (men, <383 kcal/week; women, <270 kcal/ week) were classified as having low physical activity
Slowed walking speed	Slowness was measured by averaging 3 trials of walking 15 feet at a normal pace. Individuals with a walking speed <20th percentile, adjusted for gender and height, were scored as having slow walking speed. Men met criteria if height and walk time were ≤173 cm and ≥7 s, or >173 cm and ≥6 s, respectively. Women met criteria if height and walk time were ≤159 cm and ≥7 s, or >159 cm and ≥6 s, respectively

Adapted from Ref. [6] with permission
Each criterion is scored with a 0 or 1

Data

Drey et al. investigated whether the Fried frailty criteria could serve as an inclusion criteria for a randomized controlled trial, because these criteria had usually been applied in epidemiological and very rarely in interventional studies [10]. A total of 298 people were screened: among them 181 were not frail, 116 were pre-frail and 1 was diagnosed as frail. The most prevalent criterion was exhaustion (24 % of those screened). The second most prevalent criterion was low handgrip strength (20 %). Low gait speed (8 %), low physical activity (2 %) and weight loss (2 %) had a lower prevalence. According to the Geriatric Depression Scale, 14 % of those who met the criterion 'exhaustion' were depressed. With regard to the Minnesota Leisure Time

Table 3.2 Measurement thresholds for frailty criteria according to Fried et al.

Criteria	Threshold for meeting core frailty element		Study prevalence
Exhaustion	Responds "3 or more days in the past week" to how often they felt either of the following: (1) I felt that everything I did was an effort (2) I could not get "going"		211/595 (35 %)
Weight loss	Unintentional weight loss of ≥10 lbs in past year		47/625 (7.5 %)
	Women	Men	
Physical activity	AMI <270 kcal/weak	AMI <383 kcal/weak	169/521 (32 %)
Grip strength	≤17.0 kg if BMI ≤23 kg/m² ≤17.3 kg if BMI 23–26 kg/m² ≤18.0 kg if BMI 26–29 kg/m² ≤21.0 kg if BMI ≥29 kg/m²	≤29.0 kg if BMI ≤24 kg/m² ≤30.0 kg if BMI 24–26 kg/m² ≤31.0 kg if BMI 26–28 kg/m² ≤32.0 kg if BMI >28 kg/m²	202/617 (33 %)
Walk time	≥7 s if ≤159 cm tall ≥6 s if >159 cm tall	≥7 s if ≤173 cm tall ≥6 s if >173 cm tall	249/606 (41 %)

Adapted from Singh with permission see Ref. [7]
AMI indicates activity metabolic index, *BMI* body mass index

Physical Activity Questionnaire used for the evaluation of 'physical activity', only 3 activities among the 18 selected by Fried were applicable to the studied cohort. The authors concluded, that under study conditions, good applicability of the Fried criteria was observed, however further refinement might be expedient in several criteria, especially exhaustion and physical activity in order to enhance clinical usefulness.

In a systematic review article including nine studies and encompassing 54,250 elderly patients with a mean weighted follow-up of 6.2 years, Afilalo et al. investigated the role of frailty in cardiovascular disease in community-dwelling elders [1] Table 3.3. Cardiovascular disease (CVD) was associated with an odds ratio (OR) of 2.7–4.1 for prevalent frailty and an OR of 1.5 for incident frailty in those who were not frail at baseline. Gait velocity (as a measure of frailty) was associated with an OR of 1.6 for incident CVD. In elderly patients with documented severe coronary artery disease or heart failure, the prevalence of frailty was 50–54 % and this was associated with an OR of 1.6–4.0 for all-cause mortality after the adjustment of potential confounding variables. The authors concluded, that there is a relation between frailty and CVD and that frailty may lead to CVD, just as CVD may lead to frailty. The presence of frailty results to an incremental increase in mortality, consequently implying that the role of frailty assessment in clinical practice might refine estimates of cardiovascular risk, which tend to be less accurate in the heterogenous elderly patient population.

Purser et al. tried to characterize physiological variations in hospitalized older adults with severe coronary artery disease (CAD) and evaluate the prevalence of frailty in this sample [11]. Subsequently to determine whether single-item performance measures are good indicators of multidimensional frailty and to estimate the

Table 3.3 Milestone studies to evaluate the impact and coincidence of frailty and CAD

Study	Design	n	Population	Key variables
Fried et al. [5] (2001)	Secondary analysis	450	Community dwellers	Frailty (Chin), prevalent CVD, 3-year mortality
Makary et al. [6] (2010)	Secondary analysis	4735	Community dwellers	Frailty (Fried), prevalent CVD, subclinical CVD, 7-year mortality
Singh et al. [7] (2011)	Secondary analysis	2962	Community dwellers	Frailty (Klein), prevalent CVD, 10-year mortality
Drey et al. [10] (2011)	Secondary analysis	40,657	Community dwellers	Prevalent frailty (Fried), incident frailty (Fried), prevalent CVD, 5.9-year mortality
Munoz-Mendoza et al. [9] (2011)	Secondary analysis	670	Community dwellers	Frailty (Fried), prevalent CVD, 3-year mortality
McNulty et al. [13] (2011)	Prospective cohort	1332	Outpatients with chronic heart failure	Frailty (Lachs), 12-year mortality
Gharacholou et al. [12] (2012)	Prospective cohort	309	Inpatients with severe coronary artery disease	Frailty (Fried, Rockwood, gait velocity), 6-month mortality
Purser et al. [11] (2006)	Prospective cohort	3075	Community dwellers	Frailty (gait velocity), incident CVD, 4.9- year mortality
Ekerstad et al. [14] (2011)	Prospective cohort	60	Outpatients with chronic heart failure	Frailty (Fried). 6-min walk test

Adapted from Ref. [1] with permission

CVD was defined as follows: Zutphen Elderly Men's Study, not specified: CHS, MI, angina, heart failure, revascularization, transient ischemic attack, claudication; Beaver Dam Eye Study, MI, angina, stroke; WHI-OS, any form of coronary artery disease; WHAS I and II, MI, angina, heart failure, revascularization; and HABC Study, MI, angina, coronary artery disease death, stroke. Of note, CVD was consistently driven by MI and angina, regardless of the different definitions used

MI myocardial infarction

association between frailty and 6-month mortality. In a study of 309 patients aged 70 and older, admitted to a cardiology service (70 % male, 84 % white) with minimum two-vessel CAD (determined by using cardiac catheterization), patients were examined using two standard frailty phenotypes (Composite A and Composite B), usual gait speed, grip strength, chair stands, cardiology clinical variables, and 6-month mortality. Prevalence of frailty was 27 % for Composite A versus 63 % for Composite B. Utility of single-item measures for identifying frailty was greatest for gait speed (receiver operating characteristic curve c statistic = 0.89 for Composite A, 0.70 for Composite B) followed by chair-stands (c = 0.83, 0.66) and grip strength (c = 0.78, 0.57). After adjustment, composite scores and single-item measures were individually associated with higher mortality at 6 months. Slow gait speed

(≤0.65 m/s) and poor grip strength (≤25 kg) were stronger predictors of 6-month mortality than either composite score (gait speed odds ratio (OR) = 3.8, 95 % confidence interval (CI) = 1.1–13.1; grip strength OR = 2.7, 95 % CI = 0.7–10.0; Composite A OR = 1.9, 95 % CI = 0.60–6.1; chair-stand OR = 1.5, 95 % CI = 0.5–5.1; Composite B OR = 1.3, 95 % CI = 0.3–5.2). Each tool showed a trend to an increased 6 month mortality, however only gait speed was significant.

Garacholou et al. evaluated the prevalence of frailty and its association with health status in PCI-treated patients in a sample of 629 patients ≥65 years old undergoing PCI from October 2005 through to September 2008 [12]. Frailty was characterized using the Fried criteria: weight loss >10 lbs. in the previous year, exhaustion, low physical activity, poor gait speed and poor grip strength (3 features = frail; 1 feature to 2 features = intermediate frailty; 0 feature = not frail). Health status was assessed by using the Short-Form 36 and the Seattle Angina Questionnaire (SAQ). Multivariable linear regression models were used to estimate the independent association between frailty and health status. Complete data on 545 patients demonstrated that 19 % (n = 117) were frail, 47 % (n = 298) had intermediate frailty and 21 % (n = 130) were not frail. Frail patients had more comorbidities and more frequent left main coronary artery or multivessel disease after adjustments for age and gender ($p < 0.05$ across groups) were made. Multivariable linear regression demonstrated poorer health status in frail patients compared to nonfrail patients as verified by lower Short-Form 36 scores, lower SAQ scores for physical limitation and lower SAQ scores for quality of life ($p < 0.001$ for each health status domain). In conclusion, 1/5 of older patients are frail at the time of PCI and have a greater comorbid burden, angiographic disease severity and an overall poorer health status than nonfrail adults.

A very interesting study by Mc Nulty EJ tried to identify the surgical ineligibility in patients undergoing non-emergent unprotected left main (ULM) percutaneous coronary intervention (PCI) and to assess the potential for these reasons to confound comparative effectiveness studies of coronary revascularization [13].

In 101 consecutive patients undergoing non-emergent ULM PCI, mixed methods were used to determine the prevalence of treatment selection dictated by surgical ineligibility and to establish the reasons cited for avoiding coronary artery bypass graft surgery. Mc Nulty then identified if these reasons were captured by the ACC-NCDR (American College of Cardiology-National Cardiovascular Data Registry) Cath-PCI dataset to assess the ability of this registry to account for biases in treatment selection. Finally, the association of surgical eligibility with long-term outcomes after ULM PCI was assessed. Treatment selection was dictated by surgical ineligibility in over half the ULM PCI cohort with the majority having reasons for ineligibility not captured by the ACC-NCDR. Surgical ineligibility was a significant predictor of mortality after adjustment for the following surveys: Society of Thoracic Surgeons (hazard ratio [HR]: 5.4, 95 % confidence interval [CI]: 1.2–25), EuroSCORE (European System for Cardiac Operative Risk Evaluation) (HR: 5.9, 95 %; CI: 1.3–27), or NCDR mortality scores (HR: 6.2, 95 %; CI: 1.4–27). Surgical ineligibility dictating treatment selection is common in patients undergoing non-emergent ULM PCI and occurs on the basis of risk factors not captured by the

ACC-NCDR. It is independently associated with worse long-term outcomes after adjusting for standard risk scores.

Ekerstad et al. explored the large and growing population of elderly patients with cardiovascular disease, identifying clinically relevant measures of biological age and their contribution to risk [14]. They analyzed the manner in which the variable frailty predicts short-term outcomes for elderly non-ST-segment elevation myocardial infarction patients. Patients aged ≥75 years, with diagnosed non-ST-segment elevation myocardial infarction, were included at 3 centers and clinical data including judgment of frailty were collected prospectively. Frailty was defined according to the Canadian Study of Health and Aging Clinical Frailty Scale. The impact of the comorbid conditions on risk was quantified by the coronary artery disease-specific index. From a sample of 307 patients, 149 (48.5 %) were considered frail. By multiple logistic regression, frailty was found to be strongly and independently associated with risk for the primary composite outcome: death from any cause, myocardial reinfarction, revascularization due to ischemia, hospitalization for any cause, major bleeding, stroke/transient ischemic attack and need for dialysis up to 1 month after inclusion (OR, 2.2; 95 % CI, 1.3–3.7), in-hospital mortality (OR, 4.6; 95 % CI, 1.3–16.8), and 1-month mortality (OR, 4.7; 95 % CI, 1.7–13.0). The authors concluded, that frailty is strongly and independently associated with in-hospital mortality, 1-month mortality, prolonged hospital care and the primary composite outcome. The main message of this paper was, that the combined use of frailty and comorbidity may constitute an ultimate risk prediction concept in regard to cardiovascular patients with complex needs.

Singh et al. assessed the prognostic value of frailty, comorbidity and quality of life over and above the risk factors in the Mayo Clinic risk score [7]. They examined patients ≥65 years who underwent PCI and assessed for frailty (Fried criteria), comorbidity (Charlson index) and quality of life [SF-36]. Of the 628 patients discharged [median follow-up of 35.0 months (interquartile range, 22.7–42.9)], 78 died and 72 had a myocardial infarction (MI). Three-year mortality was 28 % for frail patients and 6 % for nonfrail patients. The respective 3-year rates of death or MI were 41 % and 17 % respectively. After adjustment, frailty [hazard ratio (HR), 4.19 [95 % confidence interval] (CI), 1.85, 9.51], physical component score of the SF-36 (HR, 1.59; 95 % CI, 1.24–2.02) and comorbidity, (HR, 1.10; 95 % CI, 1.05, 1.16) were associated with mortality. Frailty was associated with mortality/MI (HR, 2.61, 1.52, 4.50). Including frailty, comorbidities and SF-36, conferred a discernible improvement to predict death and death/MI (integrated discrimination improvement, 0.027 and 0.016, and net reclassification improvement of 43 % and 18 %, respectively). The authors concluded that after PCI, frailty, comorbidity and poor quality of life are prevalent and are associated with adverse long-term outcomes. Consequently implying that their inclusion improves the discriminatory ability of the Mayo Clinic risk score, derived from routine cardiovascular risk factors (Table 3.4).

In a study, investigating frailty as predictor of outcome in patients with ACS, Graham et al. assumed, that frailty is superior to chronological age using the Edmonton Frail Scale (EFS) [15]. They assessed the EFS in a group of elderly patients with acute coronary syndrome (ACS) and administered this scale to 183 consecutive patients

Table 3.4 Unadjusted associations with the 2 follow-up end points

	Death			Death/MI		
	HR	95 % CI	P Value	HR	95 % CI	P Value
Mayo Clinic Risk Score	1.15	(1.08,1.22)	<0.001	1.10	(1.04,1.15)	<0.001
Comorbidities						
Charlson Index	1.12	(1.06,1.18)	<0.001	1.05	(1.01,1.10)	0.024
Frailty group			<0.001			<0.001
Intermediate frailty	1.90	(0.85, 4.25)	0.120	1.40	(0.84, 2.33)	0.192
Frail	5.36	(2.41,11.9)	<0.001	3.04	(1.80, 5.15)	<0.001
Health status variables			<0.001			0.032
SF-36 Mental Comp (per 10 point decrease)	1.02	(0.81,1.27)	0.893	1.09	(0.92.1.29)	0.326
SF-36 Physical Comp (per 10 point decrease)	1.72	(1.36, 2.18)	<0.001	1.24	(1.04,1.47)	0.015

MI indicates myocardial infarction, *HR* hazard ratio, *CI* confidence interval, *SF-36* Short-Form 36

with ACS aged ≥65 years admitted to a single center in Edmonton, Alberta, Canada. Scores ranged from 0 to 13. Patients with higher EFS scores were older, with more comorbidities, longer lengths of stay (EFS 0–3: mean, 7.0 days; EFS 4–6: mean, 9.7 days; and EFS ≥7: mean, 12.7 days; P=0.03), and decreased procedure benefit. Crude mortality rates at 1 year were 1.6 % for EFS 0–3, 7.7 % for EFS 4–6, and 12.7 % for EFS ≥7 (P=0.05). After adjustment for baseline risk differences using a "burden of illness" score, the hazard ratio for mortality for EFS ≥7 compared with EFS 0–3 was 3.49 (95 % confidence interval [CI], 1.08–7.61; P=0.002). The authors concluded, that the EFS is associated with increased comorbidity, longer lengths of stay, and decreased procedure benefit. Following the adjustment for burden of illness, the highest frailty category is independently associated with mortality in elderly patients with ACS. The authors warranted, that further work is needed to determine whether the use of a validated frailty instrument would better delineate medical decision making in this important, often disadvantaged population.

Makary et al. investigated criteria of frailty as predictor of surgical outcomes in surgery patients under the assumption, that preoperative risk assessment is important yet inexact in older patients because physiologic reserves are difficult to measure [6]. They conducted a study to determine, if frailty predicts surgical complications and enhances current perioperative risk models. They prospectively measured frailty in 594 patients (aged 65 years or older) presenting to a university hospital for elective surgery between July 2005 and July 2006. Frailty was classified using a validated scale (0–5) that included weakness, weight loss, exhaustion, low physical activity and slowed walking speed. Patients scoring 4–5 were classified as frail, 2–3 were intermediately frail and 0–1 were nonfrail. Main outcome measures were 30-day surgical complications, length of stay and discharge disposition. Multiple logistic regression (complications and discharge) and negative binomial regression (length of stay) were done to analyze frailty and postoperative outcome associations.

Preoperative frailty was associated with an increased risk for postoperative complications (intermediately frail: odds ratio [OR] 2.06; 95 % CI 1.18–3.60; frail: OR 2.54; 95 % CI 1.12–5.77), length of stay (intermediately frail: incidence rate ratio 1.49; 95 % CI 1.24–1.80; frail: incidence rate ratio 1.69; 95 % CI 1.28–2.23), and discharge to a skilled or assisted-living facility after previously living at home (intermediately frail: OR 3.16; 95 % CI 1.0–9.99; frail: OR 20.48; 95 % CI 5.54–75.68). Frailty improved predictive power ($p<0.01$) of each risk index (i.e. American Society of Anesthesiologists, Lee and Eagle scores). They concluded, that in surgery patients, frailty independently predicts postoperative complications, length of stay and discharge to a skilled or assisted-living facility in older surgical patients and enhances conventional risk models. Assessing frailty using a standardized definition can help patients and physicians make more informed decisions.

Stortecky et al. evaluated Multidimensional Geriatric Assessment (MGA) as predictor of mortality and major adverse cardiovascular and cerebral events (MACCE) after transcatheter aortic valve implantation (TAVI) under the assumption, that currently used global risk scores do not reliably estimate mortality and MACCE in these patients in a prospective cohort of

100 consecutive patients ≥70 years undergoing TAVI [16]. Global risk scores (Society of Thoracic Surgeons [STS] score, EuroSCORE) and MGA-based scores (cognition, nutrition, mobility, activities of daily living [ADL], and frailty index) were evaluated as predictors of all-cause mortality and MACCE 30 days and 1 year after TAVI in regression models (Table 3.5). In univariable analyses, all predictors were significantly associated with mortality and MACCE at 30 days and 1 year, except for the EuroSCORE at 30 days and instrumental ADL at 30 days and 1 year. Associations of cognitive impairment (odds ratio [OR]: 2.98, 95 % confidence interval [CI]: 1.07–8.31), malnutrition (OR: 6.72, 95 % CI: 2.04–22.17), mobility impairment (OR: 6.65, 95 % CI: 2.15–20.52), limitations in basic ADL (OR: 3.63, 95 % CI: 1.29–10.23), and frailty index (OR: 3.68, 95 % CI: 1.21–11.19) with 1-year mortality were similar compared with the STS score (OR: 5.47, 95 % CI: 1.48–20.22) and the EuroSCORE (OR: 4.02, 95 % CI: 0.86–18.70). Similar results were found for 30-day mortality and MACCE. Bivariable analysis, including STS score or EuroSCORE, suggested independent associations of MGA-based scores (e.g. OR of frailty index: 3.29, 95 % CI: 1.06–10.15, for 1-year mortality in a model including EuroSCORE). The authors concluded, that this study provides evidence that risk prediction can be improved by adding MGA-based information to global risk scores.

Conclusion

Risk assessment is the basis of any therapy, regardless of disease and age. Predicting risk in elderly patients undergoing coronary or cardiac intervention appears much more complex than in younger patients. Therefore, assessing frailty in elderly

Table 3.5 Univariable associations of global and MGA-based risk scores for the prediction of all-cause mortality and MACCE 30 days and 1 year after TAVI

	30 days after TAVI				1 year after TAVI			
	All-cause mortality		MACCE		All-cause mortality		MACCE	
	OR (95 % CI)	p value	OR (95 % CI)	p value	OR (95 % CI)	p value	OR (95 % CI)	p value
Global risk scores								
STS score								
Linear (OR per 5 % increase)	3.16 (1.24–8.06)	0.02	2.34 (0.99–5.50)	0.05	3.63 (1.71–7.71)	0.001	2.66 (1.33–5.34)	0.01
Dichotomized (≥5 % vs. <5 %)	6.14 (0.73–51.95)	0.08	8.23 (1.00–67.71)	0.04	5.47 (1.48–20.22)	0.01	3.40 (1.14–10.13)	0.03
Logistic EuroSCORE								
Linear (OR per 10 % increase)	1.32 (0.87–2.02)	0.20	1.27 (0.86–1.88)	0.23	1.79 (1.27–2.53)	0.001	1.57 (1.15–2.16)	0.01
Dichotomized (≥15 % vs. <15 %)	2.91 (0.34–24.78)	0.44	1.63 (0.32–8.17)	0.72	4.02 (0.86–18.70)	0.09	2.99 (0.81–11.04)	0.11
MGA-based risk scores								
MMSE								
Linear (OR per 3 points decrease)	2.85 (1.32–6.17)	0.01	3.67 (1.62–8.32)	0.002	2.72 (1.40–5.31)	0.003	3.04 (1.53–6.03)	0.001
Dichotomized (<27 vs. ≥27 points)	7.62 (1.44–40.19)	0.01	6.07 (1.45–25.33)	0.01	2.98 (1.07–8.31)	0.03	3.48 (1.30–9.28)	0.01
MNA								
Linear (OR per 1 point decrease)	1.30 (1.03–1.66)	0.03	1.31 (1.05–1.63)	0.02	1.27 (1.06–1.52)	0.01	1.30 (1.09–1.55)	0.004
Dichotomized (<12 vs. ≥12 points)	10.41 (1.23–88.12)	0.02	3.34 (0.81–13.77)	0.10	6.72 (2.04–22.17)	0.001	6.42 (2.14–19.31)	0.001

(continued)

Table 3.5 (continued)

	30 days after TAVI				1 year after TAVI			
	All-cause mortality		MACCE		All-cause mortality		MACCE	
	OR (95 % CI)	p value	OR (95 % CI)	p value	OR (95 % CI)	p value	OR (95 % CI)	p value
TUG								
Linear (OR per 5 s increase)	1.83 (1.10–3.05)	0.02	1.67 (1.08–2.60)	0.02	1.74 (1.24–2.45)	0.001	1.63 (1.19–2.24)	0.002
Dichotomized (≥20 vs. <20 s)	13.77 (1.62–117.01)	0.004	8.00 (1.60–40.03)	0.01	6.65 (2.15–20.52)	0.001	5.12 (1.85–14.22)	0.001
BADL								
Linear (OR per 1 point increase)	1.75 (1.01–3.02)	0.05	2.13 (1.27–3.56)	0.004	1.81 (1.16–2.84)	0.01	1.78 (1.15–2.77)	0.01
Dichotomized (≥1 point)	4.72 (1.05–21.27)	0.04	4.37 (1.13–16.87)	0.03	3.63 (1.29–10.23)	0.01	3.33 (1.24–8.95)	0.01
IADL								
Linear (OR per 1 point increase)	1.39 (0.91–2.11)	0.13	1.06 (0.70–1.62)	0.78	1.25 (0.92–1.70)	0.16	1.19 (0.88–1.59)	0.26
Dichotomized (≥1 point)	1.19 (0.27–5.31)	>0.999	0.53 (0.13–2.12)	0.48	1.52 (0.52–4.45)	0.44	1.55 (0.56–4.25)	0.40
Pre-clinical mobility disability								
Dichotomized (present or not)	5.15 (0.61–43.59)	0.14	2.92 (0.59–14.55)	0.31	3.00 (0.92–9.83)	0.07	3.86 (1.20–12.44)	0.03
Frailty index								
Linear (OR per 1 point increase)	2.18 (1.32–3.61)	0.002	1.66 (1.14–2.44)	0.01	1.80 (1.31–2.47)	<0.001	1.80 (1.33–2.45)	<0.001
Dichotomized (≥3 vs. <3 points)	8.33 (0.99–70.48)	0.03	4.78 (0.96–23.77)	0.05	3.68 (1.21–11.19)	0.02	4.89 (1.64–14.60)	0.003

Adapted from Stortecky et al. [16] with permission
CI confidence interval, *MACCE* major adverse cardiovascular and cerebral event (s), *OR* odds ratio, *TAVI* transcatheter aortic valve implantation; other abbreviations as in Table 2

patients identifies a subset of elderly patients who are at risk for adverse events (death and MI) after successful intervention.

According to Afilalo "Frailty contributes valuable prognostic insights incremental to existing risk models and assists clinicians in defining optimal care pathways for their patients."

All studies mentioned above had one thing in common, that frail patients were less aggressively managed and less likely referred for cardiac catheterization and, if treated had worse outcome and a higher risk for complications. A better understanding of frailty, when treating elderly patients seems crucial as it pertains to the care and treatment needed for the elderly. The addition of frailty, comorbidity and QOL to the usual risk assessment of elderly patients who are undergoing PCI and the reassessment of the indication may help prevent identifying those patients, who are at increased risk when receiving intervention.

References

1. Afilalo J, Alexander KP, Mack MJ, et al. Frailty assessment in the cardiovascular care of older adults. J Am Coll Cardiol. 2014;68:747–62.
2. Collard RM, Boter H, Schoevers RA, et al. Prevalence of frailty in community dwelling older persons: a systematic review. J Am Geriatr Soc. 2012;60:1487–92.
3. Afilalo J, Karunananthan S, Eisenberg MJ, et al. Role of frailty in patients with cardiovascular disease. Am J Cardiol. 2009;103:1616–21.
4. Morley JE. Frailty: diagnosis and treatment. J Nutr Health Aging. 2011;8:667–70.
5. Fried LP, Tangen CM, Walston J, et al. Frailty in older adults: evidence for a phenotype. J Gerontol A Biol Sci Med Sci. 2001;56:M146–56.
6. Makary MA, Segev DL, Pronovost PJ, et al. Frailty as a predictor of surgical outcomes in older patients. J Am Coll Surg. 2010;6:901–8.
7. Singh M, Charanjit SR, Lennon RJ, et al. Influence of frailty and health status on outcomes in patients with coronary disease undergoing percutaneous revascularization. Circ Cardiovasc Qual Outcomes. 2011;4:496–502.
8. Guralnik JM, Ferrucci L, Simonsick EM, et al. A short physical performance battery assessing lower extremity function: association with self-reported disability and prediction of mortality and nursing home admission. J Gerontol. 1994;49:m85–94.
9. Munoz-Mendoza CL, Cabanero-Martinez MJ, Millana-Calenti JC, et al. Reliability of 4-m and 6-m walking speed test in elderly people with cognitive impairment. Arch Gerontol Geriatr. 2011;52:67–70.
10. Drey M, Pfeifer K, Sieber CC, Bauer JM. The Fried frailty criteria as inclusion criteria for a randomized controlled trial: personal experience and literature review. Gerontology. 2011; 57:11–8.
11. Purser JL, Kuchibhatla MN, Fillenbaum GG, et al. Identifying frailty in hospitalized older adults with significant coronary artery disease. J Am Geriatr Soc. 2006;54:1674–81.
12. Gharacholou SM, Roger VL, Lennon RJ, et al. Comparison of frail patients versus nonfrail patients >65 years of age undergoing percutaneous coronary intervention. Am J Cardiol. 2012;109:1569–75.
13. McNulty EJ, Ng W, Spertus JA, et al. Surgical candidacy and selection biases in nonemergent left main stenting: implications for observational studies. JACC Cardiovasc Interv. 2011;9: 1020–7.

14. Ekerstad N, Swahn E, Janzon M, et al. Frailty is independently associated with short-term outcomes for elderly patients with non-ST-segment elevation myocardial infarction. Circulation. 2011;124:2397–404.
15. Graham M, Galbraith PD, O'Neill D, et al. Frailty and outcome in elderly patients with acute coronary syndrome. Can J Cardiol. 2013;29:1610–5.
16. Stortecky S, Schoenenberger AW, Moser A, et al. Evaluation of multidimensional geriatric assessment as a predictor of mortality and cardiovascular events after transcatheter aortic valve implantation. JACC Cardiovasc Interv. 2012;5:489–96.

Chapter 4
Comorbid Burden and Its Impact on Outcome

Philipp Bahrmann

Introduction

The risk of falling ill rises with increasing age. Due to the aging of the population and to advances in medical care and public health that have allowed people to live longer with incurable diseases, the number and proportion of patients with chronic diseases are growing [1]. If two or more chronic diseases exist at the same time, the state of health of the patient can be referred to as multimorbid. On average, there are five diagnoses in 65–70-year-olds, seven diagnoses in 70–80-year-olds and over eight diagnoses in 80–84-year-olds [2]. Accurate data on the prevalence of multimorbidity are available of only a few studies in Europe. A study that was conducted in several Dutch general practice centers described a prevalence of 15 % for over 60 years old patients. According to the results of a database analysis of 42 general practice centers in Germany a prevalence of 78 % was present in patients aged 80 and over. The "Seven Countries Study" described a prevalence of 10–15 % in men aged 65–84 years with different accumulation depending on the region. In Germany, 40 % of patients over 65 years had up to four diseases at the same time and over 16 % more than four diseases [3]. Because certain conditions heighten the risk of developing other conditions, patients with multimorbidity are likely to accumulate more diagnoses and experience escalating clinical complexity [4, 5].

The prevalence of multimorbidity varies by age, country and investigated patient population. The high variability in prevalence has its basis in the different definitions of multimorbidity, which were used by the researchers. However, even if the values are far apart, they show the significance of multimorbidity for healthcare

P. Bahrmann, MD, MHBA, FESC
Friedrich-Alexander-University, Institute for Biomedicine of Aging, Nürnberg, Germany
e-mail: philipp.bahrmann@fau.de

H. Rittger (ed.), *Interventional Cardiology in the Elderly*,
DOI 10.1007/978-3-319-21142-8_4

utilization and costs [6]. Approximately 80 % of spending in the national health insurance accounts for 20 % of the insured person with one or more chronic diseases [7]. In the recent analysis of the PRISCUS study, the average annual direct costs for elderly patients without multimorbidity were at 1250 € in Germany. In patients with two chronic conditions, the average annual direct costs were at € 1962 and in patients with more than ten chronic diseases even at € 6862. Therefore, the impact of multimorbidity on the social security systems are highly relevant because with an increasing number of diseases the cost of care increases predominantly linear (sometimes even exponentially) [8]. Multimorbidity is especially associated with high health care utilization and cost when it is accompanied by functional limitations. In the future, the health systems will thus face major challenges when decisions have to be made about the type of care, on the allocation of services as well as on the financing of the funding [9]. In a systematic review on the association between multimorbidity and health costs, Hodek et al. notes that the knowledge of the impact of chronic (multiple) diseases and possible combinations is of great significance to improve the care of people with multimorbidity, to use resources more efficiently and thus ultimately reduce costs [8].

Multimorbidity may also lead to polypharmacy, i.e. the administration of four or more simultaneously prescribed drugs, which in turn is a serious pharmacological problem [10]. Due to the large number of prescribed drugs the risk of adverse drug reactions increases and thus for the subsequent health care utilization in practices and clinics [11]. Multimorbidity also presents challenges in the development of guidelines and treatment recommendations, which are still largely unresolved. Clinical guidelines limit their recommendations yet often on single diseases. In clinical research, patients with multiple diseases are often excluded. Kaplan and Feinstein explained to the resulting bias: "In clinical practice, the prognostic influences of age and comorbidity are well recognized, and these influences usually receive careful consideration during the diverse decisions of clinical judgment. In statistical studies, the effects of comorbidity are generally ignored [12]."

According to de Groot et al., there are four important reasons to measure multimorbidity in studies [13]. The first reason is to be able to correct confounders, and thereby improve the internal validity of the study. A confounder is a factor that is not directly subject of the investigation. But both the intervention/exposure as well as the target size is associated with the confounder. Thus confounders could cause "confusion" in statements about the relationship between intervention/exposure and target [14]. The second reason is to be able to identify effect modification. Effect modification means the effect of a factor to a disease characterized by the presence of another factor, which means that there is an interaction between the two factors [15]. The third reason is the wish to use multimorbidity as a predictor of survival or progression of patients in studies [16]. The final reason is that a comprehensive measure for multimorbidity, which summarizes many coexisting diseases in a score, is useful for reasons of statistical efficiency.

In the literature there are a wide variety of methods to measure multimorbidity in patients. A common method is to determine the total number of diseases and the detection of chronic diseases among an underlying disease. For example, the Charlson Comorbidity Index captures both the number and severity of each disease. But a standarized procedure for the measurement of multimorbidity does not exist so far [17]. Therefore Professor Cornel Sieber, Chair of Geriatrics at the University of Erlangen-Nuremberg, criticized in a press release prior to the 118th German Internist Congress in Wiesbaden, that currently no consensus in the definition of multimorbidity and the number and type of considered diseases exists [3].

The closely interrelated concepts multimorbidity, comorbidity and frailty are defined in this capital, and then the current methods are compiled and evaluated as multimorbidity has so far been operationalized. Furthermore, the influence of the concepts will be explained on patient outcome.

Definitions

Multimorbidity

The term 'multimorbidity' first appeared in a German publication in 1976. For the next 14 years the term was restricted almost entirely to German publications. The term 'multimorbidity' used only 72 publications in their text from 1976 to 1990. Alone 66 of these 72 publications were written in German.

It was not until 1990 that concept received international attention through further research. Van den Akker defined multimorbidity, as the presence of multiple, recurrent, chronic or acute illness or symptoms within one person at the same time regardless of an underlying disease [18]. A complex structure with several individual diseases exists in multimorbidity and should always be considered as an independent phenomenon or as a specific disease state [17]. In contrast to comorbidity, there is no primary underlying disease in multimorbidity. While the term multimorbidity is structured patient-related and non-hierarchically oriented, comorbidity is disease-based and hierarchically oriented [7]. But, the terms are often used interchangeably or inconsistently in the literature [19]. As an example, a cardiologist may be concerned with the effect of comorbidity on the management of acute coronary syndromes, whereas multimorbidity captures the general complexity of patients without focusing on any single disease.

The World Health Organization (WHO) defines multimorbid patients than those who are affected by two or more medical or psychiatric conditions [6]. The intention of the WHO was to consider all the conditions of an individual that could affect the general health status. However, the term "state" is not defined clear enough for practical purposes (e.g. as whether the treated disease is a "state" in this sense) and could thus result in numerous interpretations [20].

The "European General Practice Research Network" conducted a systematic review of all relevant publications on this topic in 2011 and identified by more than 100 different definitions used by academic research. To find a comprehensive definition of multimorbidity, which is understandable and suitable for further joint research, the "European

General Practice Research Network" asked the following two questions through a study: Which of the criteria for multimorbidity can be found in scientific publications medicine and what definition can be formulated using these criteria?

The criteria found were divided into 11 topics: chronic disease, acute illness, biopsychosocial factors and somatic risk factors, coping strategies of patients, disease burden, stress the health system, disability, quality of life, frailty, social network and health consequences. The "European General Practice Research Network" finally formulated a definition of multimorbidity, which was found in the common consensus: " Multimorbidity is defined as any combination of chronic disease with at least one other disease (acute or chronic) or biopsychosocial factor (associated or not) or somatic risk factor. Any biopsychosocial factor, any somatic risk factor, the social network, the burden of diseases, the health care consumption, and the patient's coping strategies may function as modifiers (of the effects of multimorbidity). Multimorbidity may modify the health outcomes and lead to an increased disability or a decreased quality of life or frailty". This definition of "European General Practice Research Network" focused on the possible consequences of multimorbidity, such as health implications, disability, quality of life and frailty.

The above definition approaches to the definition of "geriatrics typical multimorbidity". In addition to the presence of multiple co-existing chronic diseases, the disease pattern, the temporal evolution of the disease and social factors are important. In addition, geriatrics typical syndromes are (for example, such as incontinence, confusion, risk of falls and complex pain conditions), relevant to everyday life functional limitations and disabilities of patients [21]. According to the definition of the geriatric scientific society and the health insurance companies, a "typical geriatrics multimorbidity" exists if at least two of the following 14 geriatric syndromes coexist in a patient [22]:

- immobility,
- tendency to fall and vertigo,
- cognitive impairment,
- incontinence,
- pressure ulcers,
- malnutrition,
- imbalance in fluid and electrolytes,
- depression, anxiety disorders,
- chronic pain,
- paraesthesia,
- reduced capacity,
- strong visual and hearing impairment,
- medication problems,
- high risk of complications.

This geriatric syndromes again are symptoms or consequences of various diseases. For example, a reduced capacity could be the result of heart failure, chronic obstructive pulmonary disease or cancer. Thus, these criteria are different from the commonly used definitions that focus on individual diagnoses.

Comorbidity

The concept of comorbidity was preceded by the concept of multimorbidity. In the early seventies, Feinstein defined the term comorbidity as "[...] the existence or occurrence of any distinct additional entity during the clinical course of a patient who has the index disease under study". As comorbidity he described the occurrence of an additional etiologically of the underlying disease ("index disease") independent acute or chronic illness during the clinical course. The importance and impact of comorbidity for the entire clinical course of an underlying disease, in particular their treatment, care and prognosis, was thus recognized and described already in the seventies by Feinstein [23].

A further development of the concept of comorbidity for clinical problems was done based on the number and the nature of disease, the specification of the disease diagnosis by a physician or medical history of the patient and the location of the study survey, such as general practice centers, hospitals or nursing homes, during the seventies and eighties. Indices have been developed to investigate comorbidity in clinical studies [13]. However, these indices were based on different approaches. Charlson Comorbidity Index takes into account both the number and severity of the disease, to improve the prediction of 10-year mortality [24]. The "Index of coexistent Diseases" predicts health-related quality of life after surgery, while the Kaplan-Feinstein Index assesses comorbidity in patients with diabetes mellitus [12].

However, the general transferability of indexes is restricted, as some were derived from non-representative study populations and/or the underlying data sources (surveys, databases, network of general practice centers) are not comparable. According to a summary review by de Groot et al., the necessary methodological quality criteria are sufficiently met by only four indices: the Charlson Comorbidity Index, the "Cumulative Illness Rating Scale", the "Index of Coexisting Disease" and the Kaplan-Feinstein Index [25]. Some of the above indices are used either for multimorbidity or comorbidity, depending on whether the focus is on the measurement of the total burden of disease in a patient or on the burden of comorbidities, which are in addition to an underlying disease [13]. The "Cumulative Illness Rating Scale" and Charlson Comorbidity Index are the summative indices, the Kaplan-Feinstein Index and the "Index of Coexisting Disease", however ordinal indices. Here, the final score is the highest individual score [16]. Currently there is no consensus on the best method to measure comorbidity in research and clinical practice.

The studies that collected the comorbidity in general practice centers, hospitals or groups of patients or the population of a region, investigated the resulting consequences, such as mortality, physical function limitations, quality of life, treatment complications due to drug side effects, health care utilization, quality of care and cost. While the study survey on mortality was done mainly retrospective, cross-sectional and prospective studies were available on the effect on functional status and quality of life. In Germany, the National Health Survey of 1998 raised the disease patterns of comorbidity but also their impact and consequences such as quality of life, consequential costs and health-related quality of life at the population level. In a review of 82 studies from 1993 to 1997, the analysis of causes and consequences showed that comorbidity in almost all studies had influence on different survival parameters such as mortality, functional ability, quality of life and various aspects of health care utilization [6].

Frailty

Due to demographic changes and medical progress, the number of elderly and very elderly patients will increase with multiple illnesses in all areas of care. But multimorbidity in old age is more than the sum of individual diseases. Despite the problems caused by the individual diseases, symptoms such as incontinence, cognitive deficits, immobility, such as falls, pain and other complicating factors in elderly and very elderly patients also are added (see section "Multimorbidity"). Functional limitations and disabilities arise which affect the ability of older people to cope with everyday life. Multimorbidity therefore requires a comprehensive "functional" point of view in comparison with a view focused on the disease in the elderly. It is a very interesting concept when applied to elderly and very elderly patients, since it provides a comprehensive overview of all factors that could lead to frailty.

Frailty is an independent geriatric syndrome, which describes the state of the elderly, which is characterized by the reduced load capacity to external stressors [26]. Frailty is a reduction of physiological capacity, which is not confined to one organ system, but applies across multiple systems and also is not specifically linked to a single pathogenetic process [27]. According to Schuler and Oster, frailty is a state of reduced functional reserves. Important functional reserves of the individual are reduced by physiological and pathological alterations [28]. According to Fried, chronic malnutrition leads to sarcopenia with a loss of muscle strength, walking speed and decreasing physical activity. This can result in limitations to mobility, functional ability, incontinence and increased need for assistance or even death [29].

It is a construct that is difficult to diagnose in clinical practice [30]. According to Drey, a patient is defined as frail if it has weight loss, weakness, poor stamina, slowness, i.e. low walking speed, and low activity, i.e. reduced energy consumption [31]. Finally, there is a relationship between emerging multimorbidity, which can lead to frailty and then in turn to disability [32]. Frailty, an increase in disability or a decrease in quality of life, may therefore be the consequences of multimorbidity. These are factors that make physicians aware of multimorbidity for the first time in many of their older patients.

Methods of Measurement

Summation of Chronic Diseases

Multimorbidity is commonly known as the coexistence of two or more chronic diseases that refers to the simultaneous occurrence of two or more chronic diseases in a person [18]. Previous studies on multimorbidity reported two or more diseases simultaneously in 3.6 % up to 50 % of the patients in the Netherlands [33]. Van den Bussche defined multimorbidity as the presence of three or more diseases. He was able to demonstrate multimorbidity in 62.1 % of the patients examined in primary care in Germany [34]. The comparison of these studies is difficult because of their many differences in methodology, the population and the number and type of disease. Diederichs also pointed out that the boundaries between acute and chronic disease states are often blurred, so that a sharp separation not often succeeds between acute and chronic diseases. Therefore, the methodological approach is increasingly being questioned, to measure multimorbidity with a summation of chronic diseases. Other factors as social, emotional and psychological side effects should be also recorded as the occurrence of two or more diseases in the elderly is not uncommon [17].

Also Extermann criticized that the summation of chronic diseases in the research and clinical practice is not practical. The result is a vast amount of information, if any diagnosis and their severity is considered in the patient. Therefore, in his opinion, a selection and bundling of information is required. Indices reduce all diseases and their severity to a single numerical score. Thereby, a comparison with values from other patients is possible [16]. Until now, different strategies have been used to develop indices for multimorbidity. A first strategy is the qualitative "ad hoc" selection of cases for a particular study by clinical judgment. This strategy, however, is often not systematically performed and is not very reproducible. A second strategy includes a systematic categorical description of disease occurrence by defining criteria (e.g. ICD-9 codes). This can be further refined by each disease is assessed according to their status as active/inactive and/or of its impact on the probability of survival. The Charlson Comorbidity Index (see section "Charlson Comorbidity Index") and the Kaplan-Feinstein Index (see section "Kaplan-Feinstein Index") are indices applying this second strategy. Another strategy is the bundling of diseases accordingly involved organ systems in order to evaluate them within the systems. An example of this strategy is the "Cumulative Illness Rating Scale" (see section "Cumulative illness rating scale") and the "Index of Coexisting Disease" (see section "Index of coexisting disease") [35].

Charlson Comorbidity Index

The Charlson Comorbidity Index was developed by Mary Charlson and colleagues in 1987, based on data collected from breast cancer patients. It has been used in several studies to assess the severity of existing co-morbidities and is an easy to use instrument with which the general mortality risk can be estimated efficiently. The Charlson Comorbidity Index is used to predict the relative risk of dying of comorbidity factors within 10 years [24]. In addition to mortality, there were also significant relationships of the Charlson Comorbidity Index to disability, for resumption and length of stay in hospital [13]. It is - as the name suggests - rather a method to measure comorbidity than multimorbidity. In practice, however, it is often used for detection of the latter. The Charlson Comorbidity Index contains a list of 19 diseases that can be assessed with one to six points, depending on the severity (see

Table 4.1 List of 19 contributing diseases of the "Charlson Comorbidity Index"

Clinical diseases are as follows:
Myocardial infarct, congestive heart failure, peripheral vascular disease, cerebrovascular vascular disease, dementia, chronic obstructive pulmonary disease, connective tissue disease, ulcers, mild liver disease, diabetes mellitus type 2, hemiplegia, moderate/severe renal insufficiency, diabetes with end organ damage, tumor, leukemia, lymphoma, moderate/severe hepatopathy, metastatic tumor, AIDS

Table 4.2 Weighting of the "Charlson Comorbidity Index" for 19 contributing diseases

Weighting	Comorbidity
1	Myocardial infarction, congestive heart failure, peripheral vascular disease, cerebrovascular vascular disease, dementia, chronic obstructive pulmonary disease, connective tissue disease, ulcers, mild liver disease, diabetes mellitus type 2
2	Hemiplegia, moderate/severe renal insufficiency, diabetes with end organ damage, each tumor, leukemia, lymphoma
3	Moderate/severe hepatopathy
6	Metastatic tumor, AIDS

Table 4.1). Any concomitant disease is associated depending on the risk of dying, with a score of one, two, three, or six. The score is added and the mortality rate can be predicted by the sum of the individual diseases (see Table 4.2). The research uses the Charlson Comorbidity Index in the classification of zero, one or two plus.

The Charlson Comorbidity Index has the advantage that it is very clearly structured and easy to complete, since the criteria are easy to identify and differ from each other well. An advantage is that it can be determined without patient survey, so only with the help of the medical record, and only slightly takes time for gathering and analyzing data (about 5 minutes). The index can be optionally used with and without age correction, and is validated for oncology patients. The Charlson Comorbidity Index has now been adapted to the use of administrative data (e.g. ICD-9 codes) [36, 37]. It is characterized by a very good reliability, excellent correlation with mortality and progression-free survival. The test-retest reliability, i.e. the degree of consistency of test results in the same subjects and with the same test in several testings, is good and the inter-rater reliability, i.e. the extent of the consistency of assessment results for different observers, is moderate to good [13]. A limitation of the index is that it only interrogates nineteen diseases. It does not take account of non-malignant hematological diseases (e.g. anemia).

Cumulative Illness Rating Scale

Another methodological approach to measure multimorbidity is the "Cumulative Illness Rating Scale" [38]. The "Cumulative Illness Rating Scale" aims to detect the physical deterioration of the patient by the estimated damage of 13 body systems using a five-point severity scale [25]. The "Cumulative Illness Rating Scale" was developed to assess the total medical burden and capacity for elderly patients to

Table 4.3 "Cumulative illness rating scale"

	Value 0–4
(a) Cardiac (heart only)	___
(b) Hypertension (rating is based on severity; affected systems are rated separately)	___
(c) Vascular (blood, blood vessels and cells, marrow, spleen, lymphatics)	___
(d) Respiratory (lungs, bronchi, trachea below the larynx)	___
(e) EENT (eye, ear, nose, throat, larynx)	___
(f) Upper GI (esophagus, stomach, duodenum, biliary and pancreatic trees; do no include diabetes)	___
(g) Lower GI (intestines, hernias)	___
(h) Hepatic (liver only)	___
(i) Renal (kidneys only)	___
(j) Other GU (ureters, bladder, urethra, prostate, genitals)	___
(k) Musculo-skeletal-integumentary (muscles, bone, skin)	___
(l) Neurological (brain, spinal cord, nerves; do not include dementia)	___
(m) Endocrine-Metabolic (includes diabetes, diffuse infections, infections, toxicity)	___
(n) Psychiatric/Behavioral (includes depression, anxiety, agitation, psychosis, not dementia)	___

survive and was not originally designed as a comorbidity index [16]. Miller and colleagues revised the "Cumulative Illness Rating Scale" to take account of the problems of the elderly in long-term care. In 1992, they renamed the index in "Cumulative Illness Rating Scale for Geriatrics", abbreviated CIRS-G [39]. This quantitative scale is used to detect the state of health of institutionalized frail older adults. Based on the examination of the patient and the available document, the doctor or nurses evaluate each of 14 organ systems, whether and to what extent it is affected by damage, malfunctions and activity impairment (see Table 4.3).

The 14 organ systems include heart, high blood pressure and vascular, hematopoietic and lymphatic system, lungs and respiratory tract (below the larynx), eye and ear, nose and throat medicine (eyes, ears, nose, pharynx, larynx), upper gastrointestinal tract (esophagus, stomach, duodenum, without a pancreas), the lower gastrointestinal tract (lower digestive tract, hernia), liver, gall bladder and pancreas, kidneys (without urinary tract, bladder and prostate), urogenital tract (ureters, urinary bladder, urethra, prostate, genital organs, uterus, ovaries), musculoskeletal and skin, nervous system (brain, spinal cord, nerves, and without dementia and depression), endocrine, metabolic disorders and breast disorders (including various infectious diseases and poisoning) and mental disorders (including dementia and depression). The rating is intuitive and is based on the description of the rating criteria from zero to four (see Table 4.4).

The end result of "Cumulative Illness Rating Scale" is the sum of each of the 14 individual organ systems score. The scale can vary theoretically between zero and 56 points, although a very high score is impossible because it would represent multiple organ system failures that are not compatible with life [40].

"Cumulative Illness Rating Scale" has good interrater reliability with correlation coefficients in the range from 0.55 to 0.91 [41]. The retest reliability is good [13].

Table 4.4 Weighting of 14 for "Cumulative Illness Rating Scale" contributing organ systems

Rating scale	Rating criteria
0	**No impairment to that organ/system**
1	**Mild:** Impairment does not interfere with normal activity; treatment may not be required; the prognosis is excellent
2	**Moderate:** Impairment interferes with normal activity; treatment is needed; the prognosis is good
3	**Severe:** Impairment is disabling; treatment is urgently needed; prognosis is guarded
4	**Very Serious:** Impairment is life threatening; treatment is urgent or of no avail; prognosis is grave

Table 4.5 "Index of Coexisting Disease" with its two components: "Index of Disease Severity" and "Index of Physical Impairment"

Index of disease severity	Index of physical impairment
Ischemic heart disease	Circulation
Arrhythmias	Breathing
Other heart diseases	Neurological function
Hypertension	Mental function
Cerebral vascular disease	Urinary continence
Peripheral vascular disease	Fecal continence
Diabetes mellitus	Nutrition
Respiratory diseases	Walking ability
Malignancy	Eyesight
Hepatobiliary disease	Hearing
Gastrointestinal illness	Language skills
Neurological disease	Arthritis
Hematologic disease	
HIV/AIDS	Anticoagulation

Some studies have also documented a good predictive validity for mortality and autopsy [42–44]. One study showed a significant association with the risk of hospitalization in the following year [41]. Another study reported good discriminant validity, i.e. the measurements differ from each other by different constructs [39]. "Cumulative Illness Rating Scale" is one of the few validated instruments that can be used to quantify the multimorbidity in research [45]. Before using the "Cumulative Illness Rating Scale" it should however be reviewed to what extent the design of a planned study corresponds to the original study population of the index [16].

Index of Coexisting Disease

The "Index of Coexisting Disease" was first developed in 1993 by S. Greenfield to assess comorbidity in patients with malignant tumors (see Table 4.5). Later, the "Index of Coexisting Disease" was used for other patient categories. This method helps in

Table 4.6 Weighting of the "Index of Disease Severity" [46]

Severity	"Index of disease severity"
0	No, state absent
1	Minimal or no morbidity
2	Symptomatic, active, but controlled, requires continuous treatment
3	Moderate, severe manifestations despite treatment

Table 4.7 Weighting of the "Index of Physical Impairment" [46]

Severity	"Index of Physical Impairment"
0	No significant disability, normal function
1	Mild/moderate disabilities, symptomatic, may need support for the activities of daily living
2	Serious/severe disability, symptomatic

calculating the length of stay of a patient in the hospital and the risks of repeated reception thereof in the hospital after surgery. For the assessment of comorbidity, the "Index of Coexisting Disease" evaluated separately the patient's condition by two different components: Physiological and functional properties. The first component – "Index of Disease Severity" – measures the severity of sixteen concomitant diseases, each of which is rated on a 4-point scale, with zero being the absence of disease and three indicating the most severe form of the disease (see Table 4.6).

The second component – "Index of Physical impairment" – focuses on the comorbidity caused by the functional restrictions. It assesses eleven defined functional areas with a 3-point scale, where zero means normal functionality and two repealed functionality (see Table 4.7).

Various data support the predictive validity of the "Index of Coexisting Disease". The intrarater reliability, i.e. the extent of the consistency of assessment results for the same observers, is good, while the inter-rater reliability is moderate [13]. A limitation of the "Index of Coexisting Disease" is the exclusion of psychiatric elements. Alcoholism per se is not queried by the "Index of Coexisting Disease" and an affected patient would only have positive points if he had known liver disease [16].

Kaplan-Feinstein Index

The Kaplan-Feinstein Index was developed in 1974 as a scheme for the classification of comorbidity and their prognostic relevance in terms of 5-year mortality in patients with diabetes mellitus. The index includes twelve comorbidities that may affect the long-term survival of the patient (see Table 4.8). They are each divided into four severity levels from zero (no disease) to three (severe disease). Grade three is evaluated for a state after decompensation or recently undergone life-threatening episodes caused by the respective comorbidity. Degree two describes a restriction, but not yet complete decompensation and degree one is a slight or implied decompensation or chronic disease. The Kaplan-Feinstein Index in 1986 was tested on

Table 4.8 The "Kaplan-Feinstein Index"

Items	Severity scale
1. Hypertension	Grade 0 = no decompensation of vital system
2. Cardiac system	Grade 1 = slight decompensation of vital system
3. Central nervous system	Grade 2 = impaired vital system
4. Respiratory system	Grade 3 = recent full decompensation
5. Renal	
6. Hepatic	
7. Gastrointestinal system	
8. Peripheral vascular disease	
9. Cancer	
10. Locomotor system	
11. Alcohol	
12. Misc	

patients with prostate cancer and in 1995 on patients with head and neck cancer. A correlation of limitation in overall survival was observed. Unique about this score is that it contains a weighting for each comorbidity of zero to three and the final score corresponds to the highest individual score, and not the sum of the individual ratings. The maximum score is thus three and thus comparatively low. If it is judged twice with the score two in the individual factors that endpoint number also remains at three. Meanwhile, the Kaplan-Feinstein Index for MMCI- and ACE-27 index was developed [16]. Accurate data on the validity or reliability are not known [13].

Consequences of Multimorbidity

Patients with multimorbidity have on average a lower quality of life, increased mental stress, and longer hospital stays than patients without multimorbidity. They are at heightened risk of adverse health outcomes, often beyond the effects of the individual conditions. These include death, functional limitation and disability, frailty, nursing home placement, treatment complications, and avoidable inpatient admissions. Multimorbid patients experience health care uncoordinated and evaluate the quality worse than patients without multimorbidity. The cost of health care increases exponentially with the number of diseases, in particular due to the increasing number of outpatient visits and hospitalizations. Drug treatment of multimorbid patients has other consequences: multimorbidity is counted among the strongest predictors of multi-drug/polypharmacy. It is estimated that about 6.5 % of all hospital admissions are due to adverse drug events. Since older people have a reduced tolerance for drugs, they are particularly affected.

Most treatments and practice guidelines traget a single index condition, but patients with multimorbidity are complex and heterogeneous. The traditional disease-focused approach to clinical medicine may render care that is fragmented an poorly coordinated and produce treatment plans that are inefficient, ineffective, or even harmful for patients with multimorbidity. Currently, clinicians have limited guidance or evidence on which to base care decisions for such patients.

Conclusion

This capital describes that first, there are no universal consensus on the definition of multimorbidity in the current literature. In addition, multimorbidity is often used in research and clinical practice synonymous with the term comorbidity and/or the connotations of multimorbidity and comorbidity are mixed [13]. Multimorbidity defined Van den Akker generally as the presence of multiple, recurrent, chronic or acute illness or symptoms within one person at the same time regardless of an underlying disease [18]. In particular, for specific populations such as the elderly, this definition is however insufficient because the disease pattern, the temporal development of disease, social factors but also geriatrics typical syndromes (such as incontinence, confusion, risk of falls and complex pain conditions), relevant to everyday life functional limitations and disabilities are of great importance. Frailty is a consequence of multimorbidity in these elderly patients. Many of the doctors are first made aware of the occurrence of frailty on multimorbidity in many of their older patients. The recently, in this sense revised definition of multimorbidity of the "European General Practice Research Network" moves into the center the possible consequences of multimorbidity for the patient, such as health consequences, disability, quality of life and frailty [20].

Second, there is no generally accepted "gold standard" for measuring multimorbidity. While the accumulation of chronic diseases in the research and clinical practice is not very practical because of the lack of comparability of methods and the resulting amounts of information, indexes reduce all diseases and their severity to a single numerical score, making possible a comparison with values from other patients [16]. According to a survey by de Groot only four met by the large number of available indexes sufficiently the necessary methodological quality criteria: the Charlson Comorbidity Index, the "Cumulative Illness Rating Scale", the "Index of Coexisting Disease" and the Kaplan-Feinstein Index [25].

Third, the general transferability of indices between different populations is restricted, as some were derived from non-representative study populations and/or the underlying data sources (surveys, databases, network of general practice) are not comparable with each other.

Fourth, multimorbidity is associated with poor health outcomes and significant healthcare expenditures.

The challenges of managing patients with multimorbidity are multiple, including the lack of guidelines that are applicable to these complex patients and the conflicting recommendations that arise in trying to apply guidelines developed for single disease conditions; competing and shifting patient priorities of conditions to be addressed; the risks associated with polypharmacy; and the lack of evidence on how best to treat patients with specific comorbid illnesses.

Principles of caring for patients with multimorbidity include attention to understanding a patients goal of treatment and healthcare priorities; communication between multiple providers, healthcare facilities, and caregivers involved in a patient's treatment; recognizing the potential harms associated with medical interventions and minimizing drug dosing and complexity; and identifying and addressing lifestyle and psychosocial issues that may affect the patient's quality of life and response to medial care

References

1. Nowossadeck E (2012) Demografische Alterung und Folgen für das Gesundheitswesen. In: Berlin RK-I, editor. Zahlen und Trends aus der Gesundheitsberichterstattung des Bundes: GBE kompakt. p. 1–8.
2. Hansen W. Altern und Krankheit. In: Hansen W, editor. Medizin des Alterns und des alten Menschen. Stuttgart: Schattauer Verlag; 2007. p. 10–1.
3. Aerzteblatt.de (2013) Internisten fordern mehr Forschung zu Multimorbidität. Available from: http://www.aezteblatt.de/nachrichten/49798.
4. Boyd CM, Fortin M. Future of multimorbidity research: How should understanding of multimorbidity inform health system design? Public Health Reviews 2010; 32:451.
5. von den Akker M, Buntinx F, Metsemakers JF, et al. Multimorbidity in general practice: prevalencem incidence, and determinants of co-occuring chronic and recurrent diseases. J Clin Epidemiol 1998; 51: 367.
6. Gijsen R, Hoeymans N, Schellevis F, Ruwaard D, Satariano W, van den Bos G. Causes and consequences of comorbidity: a review. J Clin Epidemiol. 2001;54(7):661–74.
7. Beyer M, Otterbach I, Erler A, Muth C, Gensichen J, Gerlach FM. Multimorbidität in der Allgemeinpraxis Teil I: Pragmatische Definition, Epidemi- ologie und Versorgungsprämissen. Z Allgemeinmed. 2007;83(9):310–5.
8. Hodek J-M, Ruhe A-K, Greiner W. Assoziation zwischen Multimorbidität und Krankheitskosten – Eine systematische Übersichtsarbeit. PharmacoEconomics German Research Articles. 2010;8(1):31–46.
9. Nagl A, Witte J, Hodeck JM, Greiner W. Relationship between multimorbidity and direct healthcare costs in an advanced elderly population. Results of the PRISCUS trial. Z Gerontol Geriatr. 2012;45(2):146–54.
10. Burkhardt H. Heterogenität und Vulnerabilität älterer Patienten. In: Wehling M, Burkhardt H, editors. Arzneimitteltherapie für Ältere. Heidelberg: Springer; 2010. p. 2–8.
11. Bahrmann P, Haack A, Sieber CC. Iatrogenität. Unerwünschte Ereignisse im Zusammenhang mit medizinischen Maßnahmen. Dtsch Med Wochenschr. 2012;136(22):1169–71.
12. Kaplan MH, Feinstein AR. The importance of classifying initial comorbidity in evaluating the outcome of diabetes mellitus. J Chronic Dis. 1974;27(7–8):387–404.
13. de Groot V, Beckerman H, Lankhorst GJ, Bouter LM. How to measure comorbidity. A critical review of available methods. J Clin Epidemiol. 2003;56(3):221–9.
14. Sauerbrei W, Blettner M. Interpretation der Ergebnisse von 2x2 Tafeln. Teil 9 der Serie zur Bewertung wissenschaftlicher Publikationen. Dtsch Ärztebl Int. 2009;106(48):795–800.
15. Ressing M, Blettner M, Klug SJ. Auswertung epidemiologischer Studien. Teil 11 der Serie zur Bewertung wissen- schaftlicher Publikationen. Dtsch Ärztebl Int. 2010;107(11):187–92.
16. Hall SF. A user's guide to selecting a comorbidity index for clinical research. J Clin Epidemiol. 2006;59(8):849–55.
17. Diedrichs C, Bartels DB, Berger K. Methodische Herausforderungen bei der Auswahl von Erkrankungen für einen standardisierten Multimorbiditätsindex. Bundesgesundheitsblatt-Gesundheitsforschung-Gesundheitsschutz. 2011;54(8):972–8.

18. van den Akker M, Buntinx F, Knottnerus JA. Comorbidity or multimorbidity: what's in a name? A review of literature. Eur J Gen Pract. 1996;2(2):65–70.
19. Fortin M, Lapointe L, Hudon C, Vanasse A. Multimorbidity is common to family practice. Is it commonly researched? Can Fam Physician. 2005;51(2):244–5.
20. Le Reste JY, Nabbe P, Manceau B, Lygidakis C, Doerr C, Lingner H, et al. The European general practice research network presents a comprehensive definition of multimorbidity in family medicine and long term care, following a systematic review of relevant literature. J Am Med Dir Assoc. 2013;14(5):319–25.
21. Nikolaus T. Gesundes Altwerden. In: Zeyfang A, Hagg-Grün U, Nikolaus T, editors. Basiswissen Medizin des Alterns und des alten Menschen. Heidelberg: Springer; 2008. p. 59–76.
22. Borchelt M, Kolb G, Lübke N, Lüttje D, Meyer A-K, Nikolaus T, et al. (2014) Abgrenzungskriterien der Geriatrie. Erarbeitet von einer gemeinsamen Arbeitsgruppe der Bundesarbeitsgemeinschaft der Klinisch-Geriatrischen Einrichtungen e.V., der Deutschen Gesellschaft für Geriatrie e.V. und der Deutschen Gesellschaft für Gerontologie und Geriatrie e.V. Available from: http://www.geriatrie-drg.de/public/docs/Abgrenzungskriterien_Geriatrie_V13_16-03-04.pdf.
23. Feinstein AR. The pre-therapeutic classification of co-morbidity in chronic disease. J Chronic Dis. 1970;23(7):455–68.
24. Charlson M, Pompei P, Ales K, MacKenzie C. A new method of classifying prognostic comorbidity in longitudinal studies: development and validation. J Chronic Dis. 1987;40(5): 373–83.
25. Glattacker M, Meixner K, Farin E, Jäckel WH. Entwicklung eines rehablitationsspezifischen Komorbiditätsscores und erste Prü- fung methodischer Gütekriterien. Physikalische Medizin Rehabilitationsmedizin Kurortmedizin. 2007;5(17):260–70.
26. Bauer JM, Sieber CC. Geriatrie 2007. Dtsch Med Wochenschr. 2007;132(25/26):1414–6.
27. Woodhouse KW, O'Mahony MS. Frailty and ageing. Age Ageing. 1997;26(4):245–6.
28. Schuler M, Oster P. Gebrechlichkeit. In: Schuler M, Oster P, editors. Geriatrie von A bis Z. Stuttgart: Schattauer Verlag; 2008. p. 102–3.
29. Fried LP, Tangen CM, Walston J, Newman AB, Hirsch C, Gottdiener J, et al. Frailty in older adults: evidence for a phenotype. J Gerontol A. 2001;56(3):M146–56.
30. Fretwell MD. Acute hospital care for frail older patients. In: Hazzard WR, Andres R, Bierman EL, Blass JP, editors. Principles of geriatric medicine and gerontology. New York: McGraw-Hill; 1990. p. 247–53.
31. Drey M, Pfeifer K, Sieber CC, Bauer JM. The fried frailty criteria as inclusion criteria for a randomized controlled trial: personal experience and literature review. Gerontology. 2011; 57(1):11–8.
32. Fried LP, Ferrucci L, Darer J, Williamson JD, Anderson G. Untangling the concepts of disability, frailty, and comorbidity: implications for improved targeting and care. J Gerontol A. 2004;59(3):255–63.
33. Schellevis FG, van der Velden J, van de Lisdonk E, van Eijk JTM, van Weel C. Comorbidity of chronic diseases in general practice. J Clin Epidemiol. 1993;46(5):469–73.
34. van den Bussche H, Scherer M. Das Verbundvorhaben "Komorbidität und Multimorbidität in der hausärztlichen Versorgung" (MultiCare). Zeitschrift für Geriatrie und Gerontologie. 2011;44(Supplement 2):73.
35. Extermann M. Measuring comorbidity in older cancer patients. Eur J Cancer. 2000; 36(4):453–71.
36. Deyo R, Cherkin D, Ciol M. Adapting a clinical comorbidity index for use with ICD-9-CM administrative databases. J Clin Epidemiol. 1992;45(6):613–9.
37. Romano P, Roos L, Jollis J. Adapting a clinical comorbidity index for use with ICD-9-CM administrative Da ta: Differing perspectives. J Clin Epidemiol. 1993;46(10):1075–9.
38. Linn BS, Linn MW, Gurel L. Cumulative illness rating scale. J Am Geriatr Soc. 1968; 16(5):622–6.

39. Miller MD, Paradis CF, Houck PR, Mazumdar S, Stack JA, Rifai AH, et al. Rating chronic medical illness burden in geropsychiatric practice and research: application of the Cumulative Illness Rating Scale. Psychiatry Res. 1992;41(3):237–48.
40. Hudon C, Fortin M, Soubhi H. Abbreviated guidelines for scoring the Cumulative Illness Rating Scale (CIRS) in family practice. J Clin Epidemiol. 2007;60(2):212.
41. Parmalee PA, Thuras PD, Katz IR, Lawton MP. Validation of the Cumulative Illness Rating Scale in a geriatric residential popul- tion. J Am Geriatr Soc. 1995;43(2):130–7.
42. Waldman E, Potter JF. A prospective evaluation of the cumulative illness rating scale. Aging Clin Exp Res. 1992;4(2):171–8.
43. Linn MW, Linn BS, Gurel L. Physical resistance in the aged. Geriatrics. 1967;22(10):134–8.
44. Conwell Y, Forbes NT, Cox C, Caine ED. Validation of a measure of physical illness burden at autopsy: the Cumulative Illness Rating Scale. J Am Geriatr Soc. 1993;41(1):38–41.
45. Hudon C, Fortin M, Vanasse A. Cumulative Illness Rating Scale was a reliable and valid index in a family practice context. J Clin Epidemiol. 2005;58(6):603–8.
46. Miskulin DC, Athienites NV, Yan G, Martin AA, Ornt DB, Kusek JW, et al. Comorbidity assessment using the Index of Coexistent Diseases in a multicenter clinical trial. Kidney Int. 2001;60(4):1498–510.

Chapter 5
Coronary Interventions in Stable Coronary Artery Disease

Harald Rittger

Introduction

Increasing age of the human population led to a rising number of cardiac interventions in the elderly [1]. Despite these trends and contrary to the well-known advantages of percutaneous coronary interventions (PCI) in elderly patients with acute coronary syndromes, there is a lack of evidence regarding the usefulness of elective PCI in elderly patients with stable coronary artery disease (CAD) as randomized controlled trials have enrolled very few patients of this age group [2, 3].

The indication to perform PCI may be different in older patients, in contrast to younger patients with higher levels of physical exercise. Lower pain levels reported for an older population [4, 5] and a reduction in physical activity, might implicate, that pain relief as the main indication for PCI does not play a major role for this patient group.

Furthermore time to onset of pain after repetitive coronary occlusions during PCI has shown to be significantly longer between elderly and younger patients with a significantly longer time to onset of pain during occlusions #2 ($p<0.001$) and occlusion #3 ($p=0.05$) [4].

The reduction of mortality, an efficacy not yet proven in an overall population, may play a minor role in an elderly population as well. Consequently alternative therapy goals like functional improvement have to be evaluated and their role defined in elderly patients.

As might be expected, the peri-interventional complication rates are higher and outcome worse for an older population in regard to the higher incidence of 3-vessel disease, a higher comorbidity and age specific changes. Therefore, a higher threshold exists to forward elderly patients to PCI [1, 6, 7].

H. Rittger, MD
Department of Internal Medicine I, Cardiology and Pneumology, Klinikum Fuerth, Fuerth, Germany
e-mail: harald.rittger@uk-erlangen.de

H. Rittger (ed.), *Interventional Cardiology in the Elderly*,
DOI 10.1007/978-3-319-21142-8_5

Contrary to patients presenting with acute coronary syndrome, with a clearly decreased mortality and a number needed to treat, which is significantly lower than in a younger patient population, the therapy goals in elderly patients with stable coronary artery disease are less well defined.

The TIME-trial, still the only trial to demonstrate the effect of an interventional therapy in an exclusively elderly population, indicated after 1 year, an outcome in favor of invasive strategy in older patients (>75 years) with stable angina, and after 4 years similar outcomes with regard to symptoms, quality of life, and death as compared to an optimized drug therapy. The invasive approach carried an increased early peri-interventional risk, while drug therapy was associated with an increased probability of later hospitalization and revascularization (TIME). However, this trial was performed in the late nineties of the last century. Therefore, the recent evolution of interventional skills and devices, as well as the introduction of new pharmacological therapies were not yet taken into consideration. Despite increased success- and lower mortality-rates for elderly patients, evidence is lacking on how the success of PCI in older patients with stable CAD is defined. Especially for elderly patients undergoing PCI for stable CAD, there is currently no suitable predictor for beneficial or harmful outcome of PCI. A comprehensive geriatric assessment may be more effective in the prediction of outcomes in older patients with CAD, as it reveals functional, cognitive and behavioral deficits. When treating older patients, it is important to identify these deficits, as they determine whether a patient can live independently or if they will be dependent on the support of another person in the future. For example, the concept of activities of daily living (ADL), is a relevant instrument to measure a person's independence in activities of daily living.

Limitations for Medical and Interventional Treatment in an Elderly Population

Generally both options, the conservative and the interventional approach, appear to be more challenging in elderly patients. On the one hand adequate dosing may not be possible due to multiple medication interactions resulting in a high risk of adverse side effects. On the other hand, elderly patients often are less suitable for any intervention than younger patients. The reason is, that this group generally appears to be sicker due to existing preconditions like hypertension, diabetes, COPD and – last but not least frailty. Vessels are smaller, more contorted and prone to complications like dissection and perforation. Furthermore CAD is more pronounced, vessels are more calcified and a higher rate of congestive heart failure in patients presenting with CAD after intervention is reported. Therefore the suboptimal results reported in the balloon era, appear to be worse in an older population, since suitability for intervention was and still is severely restricted. Due to the low evidence-level in elderly patients, a lot of discrepancies remain in clinical presentation, symptoms, diagnosis and treatment, e.g. pain sensitivity, which has been reported to be lower in an elderly population [4, 5]. Conversely others report higher CCS-levels in elderly patients, with 70 % of patients over 65 years presenting in class CCS III-IV in contrast to 50 % of younger patient cohorts [8–10].

Data on Patients Presenting with Stable CAD for PCI

When evaluating patients with stable coronary artery disease treated by intervention, there is a drop in differences found in outcome and complication rates in patients over 75 years compared to younger patients as reported earlier. This can also be noticed in ACS, albeit still counting higher adverse event rates than younger patients. Overall these rates are decreasing, probably due to an increase in skills, devices, concurrent medication and in respect to an advancement in the science of aging patients [11]. A long evolution has taken place from the earliest days of balloon intervention in elderly patients.

In the beginning of the balloon era, reported complications rates and mortality rates of up to 7 % were especially high in elderly patients [12–14]. Due to the usage of advanced materials and devices in the early nineties, the success rates were improved to approximately 90 %. Thompson et al. reported a 50 % drop in mortality rates in a comparison of 982 patients treated with angioplasty in the eighties (group A) and 786 patients between 1990 and 1992 (group B) Table 5.1. Technical success rate was 88.1 % versus 93.5 % ($p<0.001$), in-hospital death rate 3.3 % versus 1.4 % ($p=0.014$), emergency bypass surgery rate 5.5 % versus 0.65 % ($p<0.001$) and incidence of in-hospital death or myocardial infarction 6.3 % versus 3.4 % ($p<0.005$). However, intermediate-term posthospital event-free rates in hospital survivors did not decrease. The rate of death or myocardial infarction at 6 months was 4.7 % in group A versus 7.1 % in group B ($p<0.05$). Survival free of acute myocardial infarction, bypass surgery, repeat coronary angioplasty or severe angina at 1 year was 66.7 % in group A versus 54.9 % in group B ($p<0.001$).

Due to the increased use of stents, the advances in antithrombotic medications, as well as the enhanced use of peri-interventional ACT-measurement, the in-hospital mortality rate as well as long-term outcome decreased to 1.1 % and even showed a continuous improvement in the course of time [15].

In a registry recording the data of 7472 patients, an age of 85 years (without further comorbidities) was associated with a two- to threefold increase in procedure related mortality [16]. Batchelor et al. concluded, that for elective procedures, procedural risks vary widely and are strongly influenced by comorbidities such as left ventricular impairment, renal failure and diabetes mellitus. Interestingly, the authors found an increase in success rates and a 37 % reduction in cardiovascular events over a time period of 4 years, potentially outlining the rapid progress in interventional procedures.

Feldman et al., using the 2000/2001 New York State Angioplasty Registry, compared in-hospital mortality and major adverse cardiac events (MACEs; death, stroke, or coronary artery bypass grafting in emergency and elective PCI cohorts)

Table 5.1 Angiographic outcome after elective coronary intervention between 1980 and 1989 and 1990 and 1992

	Group A				Group B			
	65–69 years (n=400)	70–74 years (n=300)	≥75 years (n=282)	p value	65–69 years (n=257)	70–74 years (n=241)	≥75 years (n=270)	p value
No. of segments	578	422	421		366	339	392	
No. of vessels dilated (%)								
1	81.8	84.3	75.2		81.3	85.5	82.6	
2	17.3	14.3	23.4	0.07	17.9	14.5	16.7	0.56
3	1.0	1.3	1.4		0.8	0.0	0.7	
Success rate/segment (%)	84.6	86.5	88.8	0.16	93.7	91.5	90.8	0.31
Success rate/patient (%)	87.3	88.0	89.4	0.7	95.7	93.0	91.9	0.18
No. of grafts attempted	29	22	18	0.98	32	26	29	0.91

Adapted from Ref. [12] with permission

across different age groups (<60 years, 60–80 years and >80 years), with a large sample of 671 patients >80 years undergoing emergency procedures and 5782 patients undergoing elective PCI. Elderly patients had more comorbidities, including more extensive coronary atherosclerosis, hypertension, peripheral vascular disease, and renal insufficiency, and presented more frequently with hemodynamic instability or shock. In the emergency PCI group, in-hospital mortality (1.0 % vs 4.1 % vs 11.5 %, p <0.05) and MACEs (1.6 % vs 5.2 % vs 13.1 %, p <0.05) increased by age. In the elective PCI group, rates of in-hospital complications were considerably lower, with an incremental increase in mortality (0.1 % vs 0.4 % vs 1.1 %, p <0.05) and MACEs (0.4 % vs 0.7 % vs 1.6 %, p <0.05) in the elderly. The factor age was a strong predictive of in-hospital mortality rate for emergency and elective PCI by multivariate analysis. The authors concluded, that elective PCI in the elderly has a favorable outcome and acceptable short-term mortality rate in the stent era. Elderly patients, in particular octogenarians undergoing emergency PCI, have a substantially higher risk of in-hospital death.

The TIME trial still appears to be the milestone trial regarding the treatment of elderly patients with stable CAD [17]. In this randomized, prospective, multicenter trial, Pfisterer et al. enrolled patients aged 75 years or older with chronic angina (of at least Canadian Cardiac Society class II) despite at least two antianginal drugs. Patients were randomly assigned coronary angiography and revascularization or optimized medical therapy. The primary endpoint was quality of life after 6 months, as assessed by questionnaire and the presence of major adverse cardiac events (death, non-fatal myocardial infarction, or hospital admission for acute coronary syndrome with or without the need for revascularization). Analysis was by intention to treat. 150 patients were assigned medical therapy and 155 invasive therapy. After 6 months, angina severity decreased and measures of quality of life increased in both treatment groups; however, these improvements were significantly greater after revascularization Fig. 5.1.

Major adverse cardiac events occurred in 72 (49 %) of patients in the medical group and 29 (19 %) in the invasive group (p<0.0001). The authors concluded, that patients with angina aged 75 years or older, despite standard drug therapy, benefit more from revascularization than from optimized medical therapy in terms of symptom relief and quality of life. Subsequently, these patients should first be offered invasive assessment, regardless of their high risk profile, followed by revascularization – if feasible.

After 1 year, improvements in angina and quality of life persisted for both therapies compared with baseline, but the early difference favoring invasive therapy disappeared [17]. Among invasive therapy patients, later hospitalization with revascularization was considerably less likely (10 % vs 46 %; hazard ratio [HR], 0.19; 95 % confidence interval [CI], 0.11–0.32; P<.001). However, 1-year mortality rates (11.1 % for invasive; 8.1 % for medical; HR, 1.51; 95 % CI, 0.72–3.16; P=.28) and death or nonfatal myocardial infarction rates (17.0 % for invasive; 19.6 % for medical; HR, 0.90; 95 % CI, 0.53–1.53; P=.71) were not significantly different. The authors concluded therefore, that in contrast to differences in earlier results, 1-year outcomes in elderly patients with chronic angina are similar with regard to

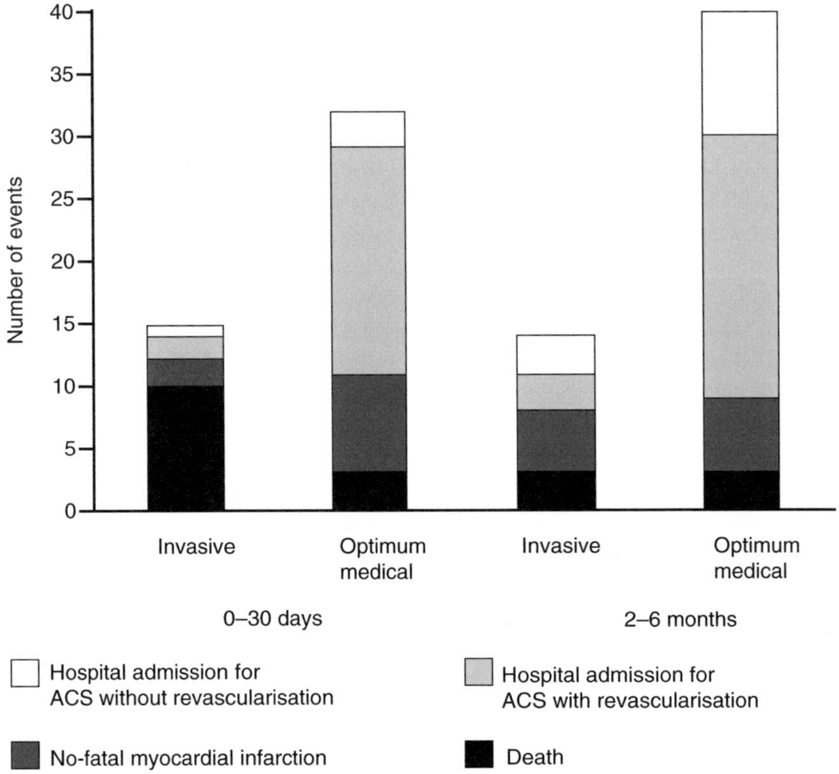

Fig. 5.1 Comparison of early and late major adverse cardiac events between medically and interventionally treated patients (Adapted from Ref. [17] with permission)

symptoms, quality of life, death or nonfatal infarction with invasive versus optimized medical strategies based on this intention-to-treat analysis. The invasive approach carried an early intervention risk, while medical management posed an almost 50 % chance of later hospitalization and revascularization.

Incorporating a 4 year follow-up of data of the survival rate of patients for invasive-strategy versus medical-strategy was 91.5 % vs. 95.9 % after 6 months, 89.5 % vs. 93.9 % after 1 year, and 70.6 % vs. 73.0 % after 4.1 years (P=NS) [17]. Mortality was independently increased in patients ≥80 years of age, with prior heart failure, an ejection fraction ≤0.45, with ≥2 comorbidities, and without revascularization within the first year. Revascularization within the first year improved survival rates in invasive-strategy (P=0.07) and medical-strategy (P<0.001) patients. The early benefit of both treatments in angina relief and QoL was maintained long term, but exemption from major events remained higher in invasive-strategy versus medical-strategy patients (39 % vs. 20 %, P<0.0001) Figure 5.2. In conclusion, long-term survival was similar for patients assigned to invasive and medical treatment.

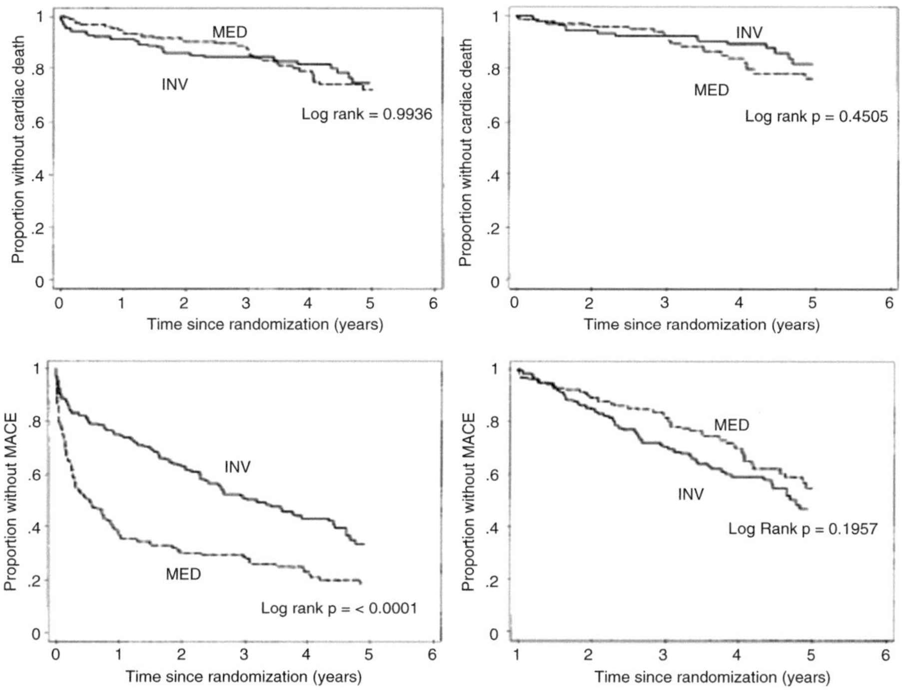

Fig. 5.2 Survival without cardiac death (*top*) and freedom from major clinical events (*bottom*) of all 301 TIME patients (*left*) and of 276 1-year survivors (*right*) (Adapted from Ref. [17])

The benefits in angina relief and improvement in quality of life were maintained in both treatments, however nonfatal events occurred more frequently in patients assigned to medical treatment. Irrespective of whether patients were catheterized initially or only after drug therapy failure, their survival rates improved if they were revascularized within the first year.

As before mentioned, this trial is currently the only randomized trial to evaluate the effects of an invasive treatment in elderly patients. The main limitation of the TIME trial is the low sample of patient numbers, which does not have the power to detect significant differences regarding "hard endpoints" like death and myocardial infarction.

A recent analysis from a German registry was based on the data of 35,534 consecutive patients undergoing elective PCI who were enrolled in the ALKK registry [18]. Of these, 27,145 (76,4 %) were <75 years, 7645 (21.5 %) between 75 and 84 years and 744 (2.1 %) patients were >85 years. Mean age was 68.5 years (60.9–74.5 years) and 25,784 (72.6 %) were male. Overall intraprocedural events were very low (1.1 %) and showed no significant difference between the three age groups (<75 years. [1.1 %]; 75–<85 years. [1.2 %];. >85 years. [0.5 %] (p=not significant)).

Rates of in-hospital death, stroke and transient ischemic attack (TIA), as well as the combined endpoint in-hospital MACCE were also very low (0.6 % vs. 0.9 % vs. 0.9 %; $p<.001$) but significantly higher in elderly patients with no further increase in the very elderly patient group. A significantly higher number of patients of the very elderly group presented with CCS class-III, with lower rates of objective signs of ischemia during exercise testing and more often no ischemia at exercise testing. Elderly patients had a significantly higher rate of severe dyspnea, congestive heart failure, anginal state CCS class III and lesions were more complex than in the younger age groups. Furthermore, elderly patients had a higher rate of reduced ejection fraction and higher rates of renal failure before intervention. However, all these disparities were not as pronounced to generate meaningful differences in outcome. Surprisingly, no differences in success rates were found, with only slight variations in mortality and overall MACE-rates. Although the medical, antithrombotic treatment still is insufficient in elderly patients (e.g. elderly still less likely receive IIb/IIIa-antagonists), this did not translate into a worse outcome. Undoubtedly, MACE-rates increased slightly with higher age, but no further increase was distinguishable from the elderly to the very elderly patient group Fig. 5.3.

Elderly patients still have a higher risk of complications, regardless of them being treated either medically or interventionally. Similar to younger patients, complications in elderly patients with an invasive approach are bleeding, renal insufficiency and longer hospitalization, which is associated with a higher mortality rate. Age is a strong predictor for postinterventional bleeding after coronary intervention. Data from the ACUITY-trial identified female gender, anemia, Heparin + GP IIb-IIIa antagonists and age as the most powerful predictors of postinterventional bleeding [19].

Furthermore, great care has to be taken in terms of the dosage of drugs. In a subgroup analysis from Protect TIMI-30 trial, dose adjustments in patients receiving Eptifibatide who had renal insufficiency prior to the intervention, lead to a significant drop in minor and major bleeding, as well as the need for transfusion [20].

Therefore, not only a careful evaluation of antithrombotic regimens is essential, but also the need for dosage adjustment of contrast agents and the elapsed time of contrast application. Many risk factors have been described for contrast induced nephropathy (CIN), however age as predictor of CIN has not clearly been identified. Among patients in the Minnesota Registry of Interventional Cardiac Procedures, CIN was diagnosed in 22 % of patients with serum creatinine >2 mg/dL and in 30 % of patients with serum creatinine >3 mg/dL [21]. The following factors have been associated with increased risk of CIN: diabetes, increased age, higher dose of contrast agent, route of contrast administration (intra-arterial versus intravenous), congestive heart failure (CHF), hypertension, periprocedural shock, baseline anemia, postprocedural drop in hematocrit, use of nephrotoxins, nonsteroidal anti-inflammatory medications, volume depletion, increased creatine kinase-MB and also the need for cardiac surgery after contrast exposure [22]. Mehran et al. have published a simple risk score of CIN, including both preprocedural and periprocedural risk factors [27]. Mehran's model includes CHF, hypotension, intra-aortic balloon pump, age >75 years, anemia, diabetes mellitus, contrast volume and an estimated

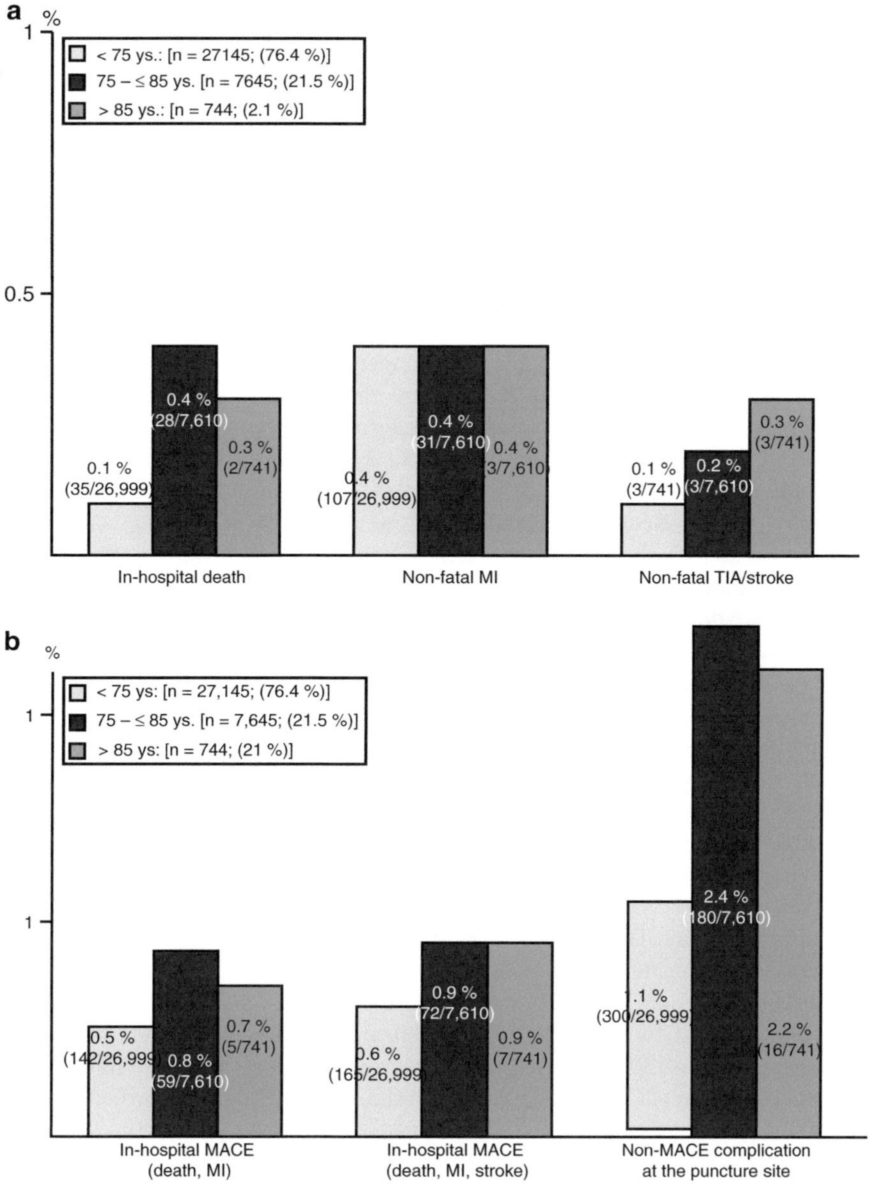

Fig. 5.3 Inhospital MACE rates according to age: (**a**) Rates of in-hospital death, nonfatal myocardial infarction and non-fatal transient attack/stroke according to age. (**b**) Rates of in-hospital major adverse cardiac events (*MACE*), major adverse cardiac and cerebrovascular events (*MACCE*) as well as non-MACCE complication at the puncture site (Ref. [19])

glomerular filtration rate (eGFR) [23]. Brown et al. have developed a similar model, however restricting it to preprocedural risks. They found that preprocedural serum creatinine, CHF, and diabetes accounted for >75 % of the predictive model, whereas other factors accounting for the remainder of the risk model were: urgent and emergency priority, preprocedural intra-aortic balloon pump use, age ≥80 years, and female gender [23, 24].

Careful assessment of the access site is crucial in terms of the emergence of postinterventional complications. Access site complications are reduced significantly in elderly patients when applying the radial approach. Hu et al. indicated in 268 elderly patients, aged between 80 and 97 years, who underwent elective PCI between May 2003 and May 2007, that the radial approach was associated with the following in comparison to the femoral approach: longer cannulation (3.0±2.8 min vs. 2.0±1.9 min, P<0.001), longer fluoroscopy time (23±15 min vs. 19±12 min, P=0.03) and higher rate of crossover to an alternative access site (9.8 % vs. 3.8 %, P=0.02) [25]. However, ambulation time (5±2 h vs. 20±4 h, P<0.001), rates of access site bleeding (2.7 % vs. 9.6 %, P=0.004), hematoma (4.5 % vs. 10.9 %, P=0.006), or any vascular complication (7.1 % vs. 23.7 %, P<0.001) were significantly reduced with the radial approach as opposed to the femoral. Multivariate regression identifies the radial approach (OR=0.25, CI=0.09–0.75) as an independent negative predictor of postprocedural vascular complications. Hu et al concluded, that PCI done via radial approach significantly reduces rates of vascular complications in high-risk populations of patients aged 80 years and older, in comparison to the femoral approach [26]. However, efficacy and procedural success rates were similar for both groups, whereas cannulation and fluoroscopy time longer and puncture failure rate higher with the radial approach in comparison to the femoral.

The most recent RIFLE-STEACS-trial randomized in an overall population, with acute ST-segment elevation acute coronary syndrome, undergoing primary/rescue percutaneous coronary intervention enhances the value of the radial access [25]. Patients were randomized to the radial (500) or femoral (501) approach at 4 high-volume centers. The primary endpoint was the 30-day rate of net adverse clinical events (NACEs), defined as a composite of the following: cardiac death, stroke, myocardial infarction, target lesion, revascularization and bleeding. Individual components of NACEs and length of hospitalization were secondary endpoints. The primary endpoint of 30-day NACEs occurred in 68 patients (13.6 %) in the radial arm and 105 patients (21.0 %) in the femoral arm (p=0.003). In particular, radial access was associated with significantly lower rates of cardiac mortality (5.2 % vs. 9.2 %, p=0.020), bleeding (7.8 % vs. 12.2 %, p=0.026), and shorter hospitalization (5 days first to third quartile range, 4–7 days vs. 6 [range, 5–8 days]; p=0.03) in comparison to the femoral access Fig. 5.4.

The authors came to the conclusion, that the radial access in patients with ST-segment elevation acute coronary syndrome is associated with significant clinical benefits, in terms of both lower morbidity and cardiac mortality. Hence, it should be the recommended approach for these patients, provided that an adequate operator and center expertise is present. Especially in an elderly population this access site should be the preferred access, facing a high bleeding rate in this patient group.

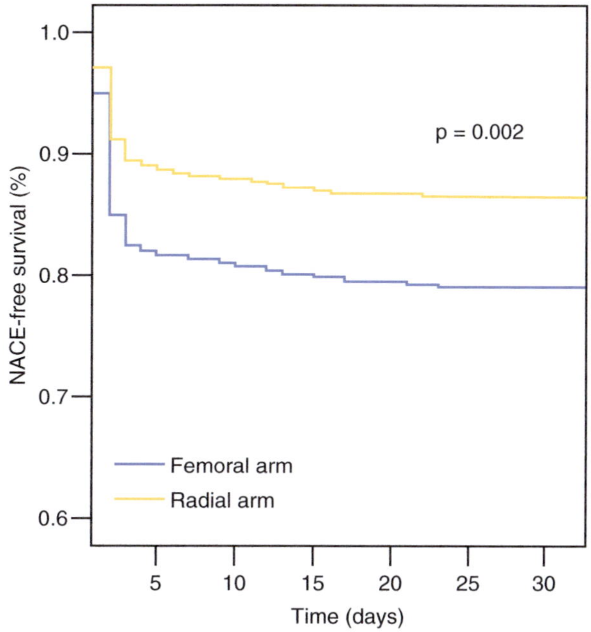

Fig. 5.4 Net adverse cardiac events as composite of cardiac death, myocardial infarction, target lesion revascularization, stroke and bleeding (Adapted from Ref. [25] with permission)

Summary

In summary, elective PCI can be performed with a high success and an acceptable complication rate in elderly and very elderly patients. Due to recent advancements in interventional techniques, success rates improved and complications were reduced especially in elderly patients. Present data confirms, that there were no or only marginal differences in success- and complication rates in elective interventional procedures found in elderly and very elderly patients, compared to a younger patient cohort. Risk factors for periprocedural complications in elderly patients are similar to those found in younger subjects. However, they are more frequent and thus the disparity in clinical symptoms still are distinctive between the age groups. The main reasons for the worse outcome in elderly patients in historical cohorts were: pathophysiologic alterations, comorbid conditions and suboptimal medication. Consequently, the reasons for the favorable results found with newer data can potentially be attributed to the advances in interventional devices such as improved performance of guide wires and catheters, as well as enhanced stent deliverability. But also the progress in interventional skills and advances in adjunctive medical therapy may be a second reason for this phenomenon.

Existing data provides evidence, that an elective PCI can be performed safely and with a high success rate even in the very elderly patient group.

However, age is still strongly predictive for in-hospital mortality, even in case of non-emergent interventions. Present data provides valuable information about the current treatment and outcome of elderly patients with stable angina pectoris.

Nevertheless, the impact of the factor age on the clinical decision making process needs further evaluation, especially in comparison of interventional treatment versus medical treatment. Generally, more attention should be paid to the elderly population in clinical research and in randomized trials, especially, as it is the fastest growing population in the western world. A randomized study would be feasible, comparing the interventional with the medical approach, but also including geriatric preconditions, like frailty, in very old patients. This ensures, that relevant outcomes of any treatment in patients with angina pectoris after 1–5 years in this patient group can be investigated. However, not only the conventional endpoints mortality and myocardial infarction have to be taken into consideration. On one hand, there is an eligibility problem for elderly patients, as several therapeutic options are less applicable for elderly patients and that these patients often are poor candidates for any procedure. On the other hand, we know that there is a different emphasis on the goals of a procedure. The indication for PCI in very elderly patients still remains questionable, since it is mainly performed for pain relief and not for a higher life expectancy. It therefore competes with medical treatment, because physical activity is reduced in this patient group. Consequently a thorough evaluation of all risk factors, which could potentially harm the patient, is of great importance. A randomized study, comparing the interventional with the medical approach, inevitably seems to be necessary in order to figure out the advantages of an interventional treatment. However, the practicability of such a study remains at least questionable, due to the limited life expectancy of this patient group.

References

1. Singh M, Peterson ED, Roe MT, et al. Trends in the association between age and in-hospital mortality after percutaneous coronary intervention: National Cardiovascular Data Registry experience. Circ Cardiovasc Interv. 2009;2:20–6.
2. Gurwitz JH, Col NF, Avorn J. the exclusion of the elderly and women from clinical trials in acute myocardial infarction. JAMA. 1992;268:1417–22.
3. Lee PY, Alexander KP, Hammill BG, Pasquali SK, Peterson ED. Representation of elderly persons and women in published randomized trials of acute coronary syndromes. JAMA. 2001;286:708–13.
4. Rittger H, Rieber J, Breithardt OA, Dücker M, Schmidt M, Abbara S, Sinha AM, Jakob A, Nölker G, Brachmann J. Influence of age on pain perception in acute myocardial ischemia: a possible cause for delayed treatment in older patients. Int J Cardiol. 2011;149:63–7.
5. Ambepitiyja G, Roberts M, Ranjadayalan K, Tallis R. Silent exertional myocardial ischemia in the elderly. A quantitative analysis of angina perceptual threshold and the influence of autonomic function. J Am Geriatr Soc. 1994;42:732–7.
6. Singh M, Lennon RJ, Holmes Jr DR, Bell MR, Rihal CS. Correlates of preprocedural complications and simple integer risk score for percutaneous coronary intervention. J Am Coll Cardiol. 2002;40:387–93.
7. Holmes Jr DR, Berger PB, Garratt KN, et al. Application of the New York State PTCA mortality model in patients undergoing stent implantation. Circulation. 2000;102:517–22.
8. Lindsay Jr J, Reddy VM, Pinnow EE, Little T, Pichard AD. Morbidity and mortality rates in elderly patients undergoing percutaneous coronary transluminal angioplasty. Am Heart J. 1994;128:697–702.

9. Claude J, Schindler C, Kuster GM, et al. Cost-effectiveness of invasive versus medical management of elderly patients with chronic symptomatic coronary artery disease. Findings of the randomized trial of invasive versus medical therapy in elderly patients with chronic angina (TIME). Eur Heart J. 2004;25:2195–203.
10. Ten Berg JM, Bal ET, Gin TJ, et al. Initial and long-term results of percutaneous transluminal coronary angioplasty in patients 75 years of age and older. Cathet Cardiovasc Diagn. 1992;26:165–70.
11. Christ M, Bertsch T, Popp S, Bahrmann P, Heppner HJ, Müller C. High-sensitivity troponin assays in the evaluation of patients with acute chest pain in the emergency department. Clin Chem Lab Med. 2011;49:1955–63.
12. Thompson RC, Holmes Jr DR, Grill DE, Mock MB, Bailey KR. Changing outcomes of angioplasty in the elderly. J Am Coll Cardiol. 1996;27:8–14.
13. Thompson RC, Holmes Jr DR, Gersh BJ, Mock MB, Bailey KR. Percutaneous transluminal coronary angioplasty in the elderly: early and long-term results. J Am Coll Cardiol. 1991;17:1245–50.
14. Bedotto JB, Rutherford BD, McConahay DR, et al. Results of multivessel percutaneous transluminal coronary angioplasty in persons aged 65 years and older. Am J Cardiol. 1991;67:1051–5.
15. Feldman DN, Gade CL, Slotwinder AJ, et al. Comparison of outcomes of percutaneous coronary interventions in patients of three age groups (<60, 60 to 80, >80 years) (from the New York State Angioplasty Registry). Am J Cardiol. 2006;98:1334–9.
16. Batchelor WB, Anstrom KJ, Muhlbaier LH, Grosswald R, Weintraub WS, O'Neill WW, Peterson ED. Contemporary outcome trends in the elderly undergoing percutaneous coronary interventions: results in 7.472 octogenarians. National Cardiovascular Network Collaboration. J Am Coll Cardiol. 2000;36:723–30.
17. The TIME Investigators. Trial of invasive versus medical therapy in elderly patients with chronic symptomatic coronary-artery disease (TIME): a randomized trial. Lancet. 2001;358:951–7.
18. Pfisterer M for the TIME investigators. Long-Term outcome in elderly patients with chronic angina managed invasively versus by optimized medical therapy. Circulation. 2004;110:1213–8.
19. Rittger H, Hochadel M, Behrens S, Hauptamnn KE, Zahn R, Mudra H, Brachmann J, Zeymer U. Interventional treatment and outcome in elderly patients with stable coronary artery disease. Results from the German ALKK registry. Herz. 2014;39:212–8.
20. Cavender MA, Rao SV, Ohman EM. Major bleeding: management and risk reduction in acute coronary syndromes. Expert Opin Pharmacother. 2008;11:1869–83.
21. Rihal CS, Textor SC, Grill DE, Berger PB, Ting HH, Best PJ, Singh M, Bell MR, Barsness GW, Mathew V, et al. Incidence and prognostic importance of acute renal failure after percutaneous coronary intervention. Circulation. 2002;105:2259–64.
22. Kagan A, Sheikh-Hamad D. Contrast-induced kidney injury: focus on modifiable risk factors and prophylactic strategies. Clin Cardiol. 2010;33:62–6.
23. Brown JR, DeVries JT, Piper WD, Robb JF, Hearne MJ, Ver Lee PM, Kellet MA, Watkins MW, Ryan TJ, Silver MT, et al. Serious renal dysfunction after percutaneous coronary interventions can be predicted. Am Heart J. 2008;155:260–6.
24. Brown JR, Thompson CA. Contrast-induced acute kidney injury: the at-risk patient and protective measures. Curr Cardiol Rep. 2010;12:440–5.
25. Romagnoli E, Biondi-Zoccai G, Sciahbasi A, et al. Radial versus femoral randomized investigation in ST-segment elevation acute coronary syndrome: the RIFLE-STEACS (radial versus femoral randomized investigation in ST-Elevation acute coronary syndrome) study. J Am Coll Cardiol. 2012;60:2481–9.
26. Hu F, Yang Y, Qiao S, et al. Comparison between radial and femoral approach for percutaneous coronary intervention in patients aged 80 years or older. J Interv Cardiol. 2012;25:513–7.
27. Mehran R, Aymong ED, Nikolsky E, Lasic Z, Iakovou I, Fahy M, Mintz GS, Lansky AJ, Moses JW, Stone GW, et al. A simple risk score for prediction of contrast-induced nephropathy after percutaneous coronary intervention: development and initial validation. J Am Coll Cardiol. 2004;44:1393–9.

Chapter 6
PCI in Elderly Patients with ACS

Harald Rittger

Introduction

While elderly patients constitute an increasing proportion of all hospitalized patients with acute coronary syndromes (ACS), advanced age itself has been identified as an important risk factor for death or recurrent myocardial infarction (MI) in this setting [1]. However, the use of invasive diagnostic and therapeutic procedures decreases with increasing age. Presumably due to the fear of complications and in combination with an uncertainty about the possible success of such an intervention [2–8]. Subsequently, elderly patients with ACS have often been treated conservatively, despite increasing evidence that patients with more advanced disease and comorbidities (as typically observed in an elderly population) may actually gain most from an interventional coronary revascularization approach (e.g. percutaneous coronary intervention, PCI) [2, 3].

Only very recent observations, that elderly patients have the potential for the highest benefit from an interventional approach, lowered the threshold to consider aggressive revascularization strategies in this particular patient group [5]. However up to now, it is not known, how far this evidence guides the decision making process in physicians warranting immediate decisions on the different management strategies in this complex patient group, which may affect short- and long term outcome.

As specific evidence is lacking for this patient group and in light of a completely occluded artery in elderly patients presenting with ST-elevation myocardial infarction (STEMI)-ACS, for the majority of cases no different treatment is justified in comparison to younger patients Fig. 6.1.

H. Rittger, MD
Department of Internal Medicine I, Cardiology and Pneumology, Klinikum Fuerth, Fuerth, Germany
e-mail: harald.rittger@uk-erlangen.de

H. Rittger (ed.), *Interventional Cardiology in the Elderly*,
DOI 10.1007/978-3-319-21142-8_6

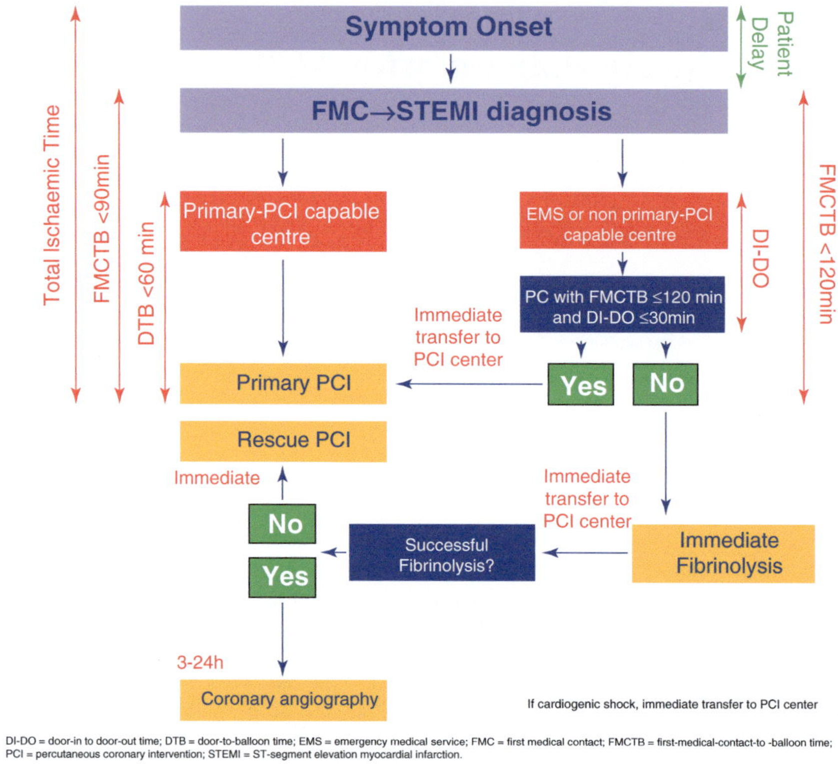

Fig. 6.1 Organization of STEMI patients, describing pre- and in-hospital management and reperfusion strategies. Care should be given to anticoagulative therapies, but also individual therapy disposals are of high importance. Despite a higher bleeding rate with anticoagulation and especially fibrinolysis, no different treatment in elderly patients is warranted *DI-DO* door-in to door-out time, *DTB* door-to-balloon time, *EMS* emergency medical service, *FMC* first medical contact, *FMCTB* first-medical-contact-to-balloon time, *PCI* percutaneous coronary intervention, *STEMI* ST-segment elevation myocardial infarction (Adapted from Windecker et al. with permission. (see Ref. [9]))

Nevertheless, with increasing age the incidence of STEMI-ACS decreases, and to some extent more patients present with NSTEMI-ACS (non ST-elevation myocardial infarction). In NSTEMI-ACS the situation appears to be more complex. Patients often have multiple comorbidities and diffuse coronary artery disease without the possibility to identify a culprit lesion. The higher complication rate for elderly patients treated interventionally additionally impedes the decision to perform intervention in NSTEMI-ACS. Specific patients are often denied interventional treatment, while other patients with a possibly higher risk for complications, receive an invasive treatment. Although strong evidence [10] exists that high risk subsets, i.e. elderly patients, may actually gain most from an intervention, there is an obvious lack of evidence, since patients >75 years comprise only 9 % of clinical trial population and only about 50 % of registry patients [9]. In the past, presumably due to the fear of complications and in combination with an ambiguity concerning the success of an intervention, decisions resulted in a reluctance to perform invasive procedures in elderly patients.

Despite all advances and increasing evidence, treatment decisions in elderly patients with NSTEMI are characterized by a continuing uncertainty about the following:

- the adequate type and
- the adequate time of treatment (for those patients who are considered for invasive treatment; e.g. interventional versus conservative with optimal medical therapy, need for pre-interventional preparation [recompensation, hydration, respiratory stabilization])
- the adequate risk assessment to identify patients who will benefit from an intervention and those, who will not
- the adequate outcome measurement of any treatment in elderly patients (mortality and MI versus improvement in functional capacity).

Data

There is limited randomized trial data available to guide treatment in elderly patients with acute coronary syndromes. In a recent large German multicenter registry, substantial age related differences were identified in the diagnosis and treatment of elderly patients presenting to a hospital with acute myocardial infarction. The results confirmed, that elderly patients are a significant and increasing proportion of the total population treated for ACS [11–13]. The proportion of 28.1 % elderly patients in the more recent ALKK registry data of 2008 is 2.4 % higher than the numbers enrolled in the older "Global Registry of Acute Coronary Events" (GRACE)–registry, which included 24,165 patients with a rate of 25.7 % subjects aged >75 years, possibly suggesting an increase over time [11].

In a prior published registry of patients with NSTEMI-ACS, over 35 % of the population were >75 years, emphasizing the growing importance to examine outcomes in the older age group [14]. In contrast to a significant difference in treatment modalities between elderly and younger patients (invasive strategy 39 % vs. 56 % with a 30-day mortality nearly fourfold higher in the elderly population) the study identified, that age-related differences in diagnostics or the percentage of patients who were treated with PCI in comparison to the younger patient cohort, were much less pronounced. Therefore, the more recent data showed a trend towards a stronger adherence to evidence based medicine with increased utilization of resources in elderly patients albeit the recommendations were primarily based on younger cohorts.

As outlined before, older patients with suspected acute myocardial infarction (MI) often present to the emergency department (ED) with atypical symptoms and inconclusive electrocardiograms (ECG). The use of cardiac Troponin (cTn) has considerably improved risk assessment and diagnostic accuracy in the ED. The diagnosis of MI has been further improved by the introduction of novel high-sensitivity cTn assays. Their analytical precision can lower the cTn cut-off point, according to current definition of

Table 6.1 Criteria for patients at high risk with urgent indication for an invasive management

Primary criteria
1. Relevant rise or fall in troponin
2. Dynamic ST- or T-wave changes (symptomatic or silent)
3. GRACE score >140
Secondary criteria
4. Diabetes mellitus
5. Renal insufficiency (eGFR <60 mL/min/1.73 m^2)
6. Reduced LV function (ejection fraction <40 %)
7. Early post-infarction angina
8. Recent PCI
9. Prior CABG
10. Intermediate to high GRACE risk score (http://www.gracescore.org)

Adapted from Windecker et al. with permission (see Ref. [9])
CABG coronary artery bypass grafting, *eGFR* estimated glomerular filtration rate, *GRACE* Global Registry of Acute Coronary Events, *LV* left ventricular, *PCI* percutaneous coronary intervention

acute MI (cut-off defined as the 99 % confidence interval of a healthy reference population). These assays can measure low-level myocardial injury, which are not detectable by standard cTn assays. However, Bahrmann et al. showed that the introduction of high-sensitivity cTn assays substantially increases sensitivity to identify older patients with ACS, even at the time of presentation to the emergency department at the cost of specificity. Subsequently, the prevalence of elevated cTn has more than doubled with the use of high-sensitivity cTn in older patients. No coronary cause was found in two-thirds of older patients, although more non-ST-elevation myocardial infarction (NSTEMI) patients were diagnosed earlier by high-sensitivity cTn [15]. Therefore, the emergency physician encounters increasing difficulties to identify those patients who are in need for invasive diagnostics [16]. In this setting, the use of an additional marker, for instance copeptin, may be helpful for diagnostic work-up. Copeptin is the stable signal peptide of the vasopressin precursor and is considered as a non-specific marker of stress. Bahrmann et al. showed that the diagnostic improvement of copeptin in addition to high-sensitivity cTn is moderate, but it may help to reliably rule out NSTEMI in unselected older patients presenting to the ED [17]. In older patients serial high-sensitivity cTn measurements and absolute delta-changes at 3 h were more valuable for early diagnosis of NSTEMI [18].

On the basis of evidence from randomized trials, which were predominately performed in younger patients, guidelines recommend early interventional treatment for high-risk patients in the presence of ACS [9]. In recent years increasing evidence has suggested, that patients at risk, including elderly patients, gain most from invasive procedures in the presence of ACS [10, 11, 19]. The extent to which this evidence has had an impact on real world management of elderly patients with ACS remains unclear. Elderly patients with ACS, a high risk population itself, often do not undergo interventional treatment as recommended by current guidelines [11, 20] Table 6.1.

In a study, evaluating treatment decisions in elderly patients with NSTEMI-ACS Rittger et al. found, that age itself was the most powerful predictor of conservative treatment in a population of elderly patients presenting with ACS to the hospital [21]. This finding was very much in accordance with previous reports. In a registry of patients with NSTEMI a significant difference was found in the treatment modalities between elderly and younger patients (invasive approach 39 % vs. 56 %) and outcome with a 30-day mortality was nearly 4-fold higher in the elderly patients [14]. Comparably, in the GRACE registry, in which elderly (n=4776; 19.8 %) and very elderly (n=1427; 5.9 %) were diagnosed with coronary angiography in only 55 % of the cases and 33 % respectively, while 67 % of the younger patient population received coronary angiography [11].

In the previous mentioned report of Rittger et al., the second most important factors to influence decision making, were Killip Class III and the presence of multivessel disease. The reluctance in forwarding patients with Killip Class III to an invasive/interventional treatment might be explained by the apprehension towards mechanical ventilation combined with a prolonged stay in the intensive care unit. Both potential consequences of the deterioration of the respiratory situation due to the use of contrast agents and a prolonged intervention time. This is emphasized by the fact, that patients with Killip Class II were more likely to be treated interventionally and that the presence of Killip Class IV (patients in cardiogenic shock) had no significant impact on the treatment strategy.

Impending renal failure explains adequately, why an interventional approach is delayed or withheld. Nevertheless, in a recent analysis, Morici et al. could identify, by evaluating the association between baseline creatinine clearance (CrCl), coronary revascularization during index admission and 1-year mortality in elderly patients with an acute coronary syndrome (ACS), that coronary revascularization decreases the risk of 1-year death across each CrCl category and is one of the most powerful predictors of 1-year outcome. The authors stratified 313 patients aged ≥75 into four groups, according to CrCl on admission (using a cutoff of 45 ml/min) and coronary revascularization versus medical management. The mean age of the study population was 81 years and the median serum creatinine level on admission was 1.0 mg/dl (interquartile range (IQR) 0.8–1.3). Patients with impaired renal function treated medically had a higher in-hospital and 1-year mortality rate, especially if compared with patients with preserved renal function undergoing revascularization (1-year mortality 22.9 % versus 4.9 %). Across the spectrum of CrCl categories, coronary revascularization was independently associated with a lower risk of mortality (HR 0.405; 95 % CI 0.174–0.940; p=0.035). The authors concluded, that coronary revascularization decreases the risk of 1-year mortality across each CrCl category and is one of the most powerful predictors of 1-year outcome [22].

Patient selection appears to be the most crucial point – choosing patients in an elderly population who will benefit most from coronary intervention. Conditions like the presence of a prior stroke or obesity, the fear of intracranial hemorrhage or access site complications, may deter the responsible physician to forward these patients to coronary angiography and PCI. The type of myocardial infarction (NSTEMI or STEMI) or the presence of prior AMI, as well as the presence of supraventricular arrhythmias has less, but still significant, influence on the treatment strategy. It is comprehensible, that an acute invasive intervention is denied to elderly patients presenting with tachyarrhythmic atrial fibrillation. However, according to current data, the presence of prior AMI bears a tremendous risk and such a patient should be forwarded to intervention as soon as possible. Interestingly, a prior CABG procedure and the presence of COLD seems to have less influence on the treatment decision [21].

The observation in the above mentioned study, that survival is significantly worse in conservatively treated patients who did not undergo invasive coronary angiography and PCI, as well as the significantly higher in-hospital and long-term mortality rate for those patients, is a well established finding in interventional cardiology. Although overall interventional success rates in this study were relatively low, compared to a younger patient cohort, this did not forestall a highly significant better outcome for those patients, who were treated interventionally.

This phenomenon is best described as "therapeutical paradoxon": patients with the highest risk of complications gain the greatest benefit from the intervention. There are numerous examples for this phenomenon. In the prior mentioned GRACE registry, total in-hospital mortality was 15.6 % in the conservatively treated group and as low as 3.5 % in the interventionally treated group [11]. Morrison et al. reported a 30-day survival of 87 % in 131 patients presenting with ACS receiving angioplasty with unstable angina [19]. In another study Munoz and co. reported in 76 patients >75 years, predominantly with unstable angina, an in-hospital mortality rate of 6.6 % [23]. In a recent analysis, Bauer et al. investigated the impact of an invasive treatment in elderly patients presenting with NSTEMI. They analyzed data of elderly patients (≥75 years) with NSTEMI, who were enrolled in the German Acute Coronary Syndromes registry between July 2000 and November 2002. Overall, the 1936 patients were divided into two groups: 1005 (51.9 %) underwent coronary angiography and/or revascularization, 931 (48.1 %) received conservative treatment. In the invasive group, percutaneous coronary intervention was performed in 37.5 % within 48 h and in 17.6 % after 48 h, whereas 9.8 % underwent coronary artery bypass grafting during hospitalization. In-hospital death (12.5 % vs. 6.0 %, $P<0.0001$) and death/myocardial infarction (17.3 % vs. 9.6 %, $P<0.0001$) occurred significantly less often in patients with invasive strategy. After adjustment of the confounding factors in the propensity score analysis, the invasive strategy remained superior for mortality (OR 0.55, 95 % CI 0.35–0.86) and death and non-fatal myocardial infarction (OR 0.51, 95 % CI 0.35–0.75) and 1 year mortality (OR 0.56, 95 % CI 0.38–0.81). Major bleeding complications tended to be more frequent in the invasive group (8.8 % vs. 5.8 %, $P=0.07$). The authors concluded that in clinical practice, elderly patients with NSTEMI, an invasive strategy was associated with improved in-hospital and 1 year outcome, however with a trend towards more bleeding complications [24] Fig. 6.2.

The post hoc analysis of the TACTICS-TIMI-18 trial showed, that an early invasive strategy can significantly improve outcomes among elderly patients with non-ST segment elevation MI. After 6 months, mortality was 10.8 % for invasively treated patients and 21.6 % in conservatively treated patients [10]. Since inclusion

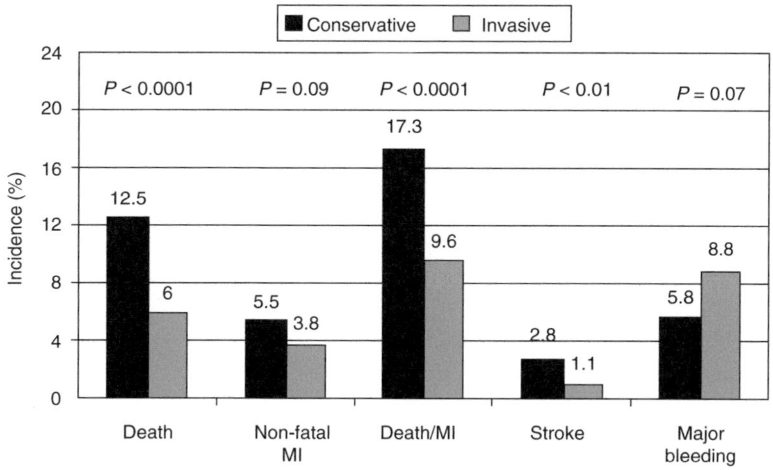

Fig. 6.2 Effectiveness of invasive vs. conservative treatment in patients presenting with ACS (Adapted from Bauer et al. with permission (see Ref. [26]))

was limited to restrictive in- and exclusion criteria, patients with excess comorbidities were excluded. This is an important fact, as the results of the randomized trials, which are not specifically designed for elderly, cannot be transferred to clinical practice especially in this heterogeneous patient group. On the other hand, a high comorbid burden may have also prevented the inclusion of those patients in registries.

Regarding patient selection and triage to one of the two treatment modalities, none of the registries investigated the reasons for the reluctance to forward patients to interventional procedures (Fig. 6.3).

As already mentioned, one of the main concerns not to forward patients to intervention is advanced age. This reluctance is probably based on the fear of complications, which are known to occur predominately in elderly patients. Summarizing the above mentioned results, it seems, that in-hospital mortality in ACS in the elderly is not only a reflection of the natural history of the disease or a consequence of intraprocedural complications, but rather a result of treatment choice, a decision made mainly by the treating physician. Nevertheless several analyses performed recently, showed that these complication rates are declining [25]. In the above mentioned analysis, besides mortality, complication rates were not significantly different in interventionally and conservatively treated patients. There was a trend to a higher risk of major bleeding, but bleeding was noted in both, interventionally and conservatively treated patients [21]. These findings are similar to the analysis of Bauer et al., who identified higher bleeding rates in intervened elderly patients, however these results were not significant [24].

In the above mentioned recent German registry, comparing outcomes in patients treated with ACS, complication rates were threefold higher in very elderly patients. Nonetheless, although primary success rates were worse, the number of AEs in the

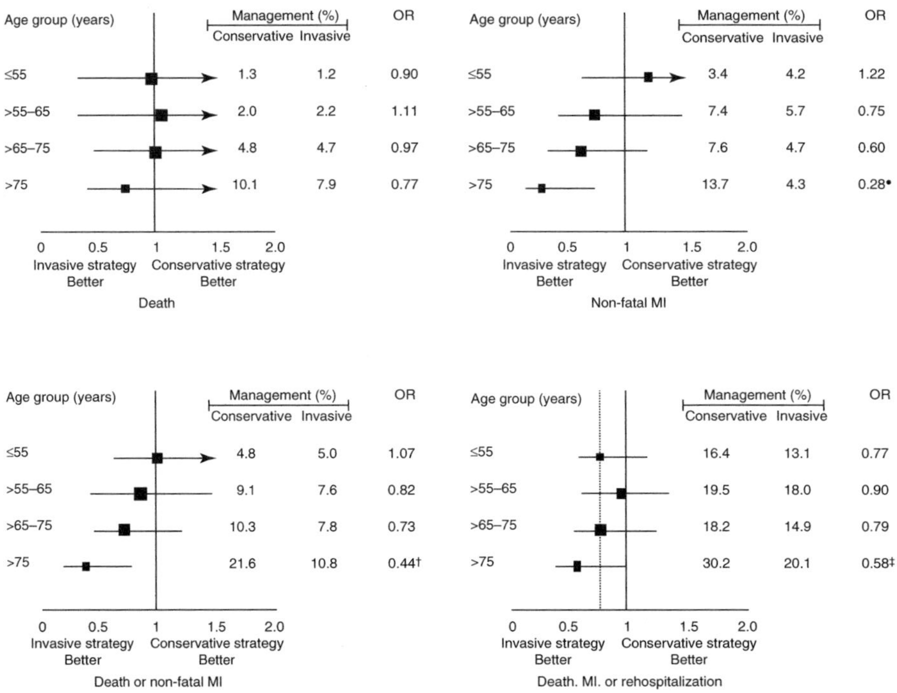

Fig. 6.3 "Therapeutical paradox", showing the clear benefit for elderly patients regarding the endpoints death, non-fatal MI and rehospitalization (Adapted from Bach et al. with permission (see Ref. [10]))

elderly remained in a range, which is concordant with the literature. Consequently the benefits gained from intervention outweighed the complications [4, 10, 14, 23].

Despite technical advances in recent years, percutaneous revascularization in the elderly still has a relatively high mortality rate, primarily due to increased multimorbidity as an inherent consequence of advanced age and secondarily as a consequence of a greater prevalence of multivessel disease and depressed left ventricular function.

The success of a certain procedure is always dependent from the health status of the individual undergoing the procedure. While health status across individuals of a young age cohort is rather homogenous, biological diversity increases with age. This is probably the main reason, why risk scores used for younger patients, such as the Global Registry of Acute Coronary Events (GRACE)-Risk-Score, seems to be less predictive in older patients.

The large multinational observational global registry of acute coronary events (GRACE) has been used to derive regression models to predict death in hospital and death after discharge in patients with acute coronary syndrome [11] Fig. 6.4. However, since age is a major risk factor in this model and part of the risk score itself, the value of this score for the prediction of adverse events seems less valuable

Risk calculator for 6-Month Postdischarge Mortality Alter Hospitalization lor Acute Coronary Syndrome

Record the points for each variable at the bottom left and sum the points to calculate the total risk score. Find the total score on the x-axis of the nomogram plot. The corresponding probability on the y-axis is the estimated probability of all-cause mortality from hospital discharge to 6 months.

Medical History

① Age in Years — Points

Age in Years	Points
≤29	0
30–39	0
40–49	18
50–59	36
60–69	55
70–79	73
80–89	91
≥90	100

② History of Congestive Heart Failure — 24

③ History of Myocardial Infarction —

Findings at Initial Hospital Presentation

④ Resting Heart Rate, beats/min — Points

Resting Heart Rate, beats/min	Points
≤49.9	0
50–69.9	3
70–89.9	9
90–109.9	14
110–149.9	23
150–199.9	35
≥200	43

⑤ Systolic Blood l'ressu'e, mmHg

Systolic Blood Pressure, mmHg	Points
≤79.9	24
80–99.9	22
100–119.9	18
120–139.9	14
140–159.9	10
160–199.9	4
≥200	0

1

⑥ ST-segment Depression — 11

Findings During Hospitalization

⑦ Initial Serum Creatinine, mg/dL — Points

Initial Serum Creatinine, mg/dL	Points
0–0.39	1
0.4–0.79	3
0.8–1.19	5
1.2–1.59	7
1.6–1.99	9
2–3.99	15
≥4	20

⑧ Elevated Cardiac Enzymes — 15

⑧ Elevated Cardiac Enzymes Percutaneous Coronary Invervention — 14

Points

① ______
② ______
③ ______
④ ______
⑤ ______
⑥ ______
⑦ ______
⑧ ______
⑨ ______

Total Risk Score ______ (Sum of points)

Mortality Risk ______ (From Plot)

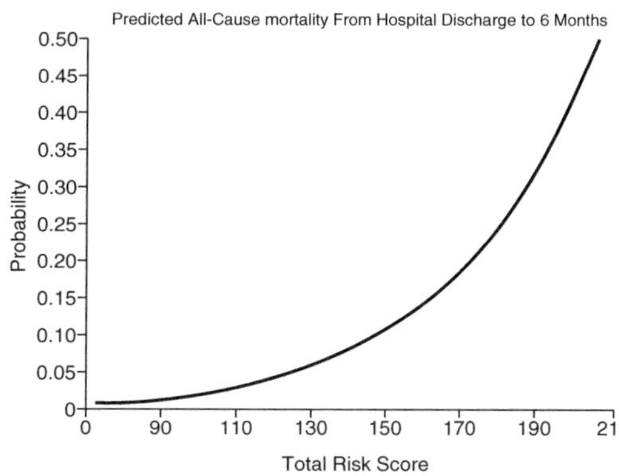

Fig. 6.4 Risk calculator for 6 months mortality after hospitalization for acute coronary syndrome (GRACE-Score) (www.gracescore.co.uk)

in elderly patients. Using the GRACE risk score mortality can best be described as follows: f(x) = (1/(1 + (exp−(−7.966 + (0.031*x)))))*100. In a retrospective study of 1001 patients >75 years, mean GRACE risk score in patients treated conservatively was 168,87, and 150,24 in patients treated interventionally. Attributed mortality risk according to this calculation was 10.22 % for the non-invasive group and 3.53 % for the invasive group. The observed mortality was 20.2 % for the conservatively and 2.4 % for the invasively treated patients [21].

Another study, using the EURO-score (European System for Cardiac Operative Risk Evaluation), evaluated characteristics and outcomes of elderly patients undergoing isolated AVR. All patients were aged 80 years or older ($n = 282$). Patient age was 82 ± 2 years (low risk), 82.7 ± 2.7 years (moderate risk), and 83.6 ± 3.1 years (high risk), respectively ($p < 0.05$). Mean ES(log) predicted risk of mortality was 7.3 ± 1.4 % (low risk), 13.7 ± 2.5 % (moderate risk), and 33.0 ± 11.5 % (high risk; $p < 0.05$). The observed mortality was 7.5 % (low risk), 12.6 % (moderate risk), and 12.5 % (high risk; $p = 0.4$). The authors concluded, that EURO-score risk stratification is imprecise for the prediction of perioperative mortality among octogenarian AVR patients, but may be useful for predicting mortality during medium-term follow-up [26].

In a prospective cohort study, Schoenenberger et al. showed that older patients across the whole spectrum of ACS were less likely to receive guideline-recommended therapies, even after adequate adjustment for comorbidities. They determined that the prognosis of older patients with ACS may be improved by increased adherence to guideline-recommended medical and interventional therapies [27]. In two more recent studies, Schoenenberger aimed to assess mortality and functional development in elderly patients undergoing transcatheter aortic valve implantation (TAVI) and to identify predictors of mortality and functional decline. Over a 6-month period, functional status worsened only in a minority of patients surviving TAVI. The frailty index, but not the established risk scores, was predictive of functional decline [28].

Evaluating patients with stable coronary artery disease, decreasing differences are to be found in outcome and complication rates in patients >75 years, compared with previous reports. Even in ACS, albeit still counting higher adverse event rates compared to younger patients, these rates are overall decreasing. Probably due to developing skills, improvement of devices, concurrent medication and presumably in respect to the increasing body of knowledge of aging patients, for instance decreasing pain sensitivity. Comparing the outcome of older versus younger patients with CABG-procedure in a series of 300 patients with left main disease Rittger et al. showed, that there was no difference in outcome and quality of life between older and younger patients treated with PCI [29]. In light of these results, a special risk score including elderly patients should be developed. This stratification should aim to identify elderly patients with ACS, who are suitable for reperfusion therapy, with the largest survival benefit.

Very limited randomized data is available concerning the treatment of very elderly patients with ACS. In the Italian elderly ACS study, Savonitto et al. evaluated the risk versus benefit ratio of an early aggressive (EA) approach in elderly patients with non-ST-segment elevation acute coronary syndromes (NSTEACS) [30]. A total of 313 patients ≥75 years of age (mean 82 years) with NSTEACS, within 48 h from qualifying symptoms, were randomly allocated to an EA strategy (coronary angiography and when indicated, revascularization within 72 h) or an initially conservative (IC) strategy (angiography and revascularization only for recurrent ischemia). The primary endpoint was the composite of death, myocardial infarction, disabling stroke and repeat hospital stay for cardiovascular causes or severe bleeding within 1 year. During admission, 88 % of the patients in the EA

Table 6.2 Cumulative rates of the composite primary endpoint in the Italian elderly study

Outcome	EA (n=154)	IC (n=159)	HR (95 % CI)	Log-rank p value
Primary composite endpoint	43 (27.9 %)	55 (34.6 %)	0.80 (053–1.19)	0.26
Death	19 (12.3)	22 (13.8)	0.87 (0.49–156)	0.65
Cardiovascular	16 (10.4)	17 (10.7)		
Noncardiovascular	3 (2.0)	4 (2.5)		
Unknown	—	1 (0.6)		
Myocardial infarction	11 (7.1)	17 (10.7)	0.67 (0.33–1.36)	037
Death + myocardial infarction	28 (18.2)	34 (21.4)	0.85 (052–1.41)	053
Disabling stroke	0	0		
Repeat hospital stays for				
CV causes or severe bleeding	18 (11.7)	22 (13.8)	0.81 (0.45–1.46)	0.49
Cardiovascular causes	16 (10.4)	21 (13.2)		
Severe recurrent ischemia	0	4 (25)		
Revascularization	5 (3.3)	9 (5.7)		
Heart failure	7 (4.6)	4 (25)		
Non-CNS embolism	0	1 (0.6)		
Cardiac arrhythmia	4 (2.6)	3 (1.9)		
Severe bleeding[a]	2 (1.3)	1 (0.6)		
Noncardiovascular causes	8 (5.2)	5 (33)		

Adapted from Ref. [30] with permission
Values are n (%)
CI confidence interval, *CV* cardiovascular, *HR* hazard ratio; other abbreviations as in Tables 1 and 5
[a]Bleeding Academic Research Consortium grades 2, 3a, and 3b.

group underwent angiography (55 % revascularization), compared with 29 % (23 % revascularization) in the IC group. The primary outcome occurred in 43 patients (27.9 %) in the EA group and 55 (34.6 %) in the IC group (hazard ratio [HR]: 0.80; 95 % confidence interval [CI]: 0.53–1.19; p=0.26). The rates of mortality (HR: 0.87; 95 % CI: 0.49–1.56), myocardial infarction (HR: 0.67; 95 % CI: 0.33–1.36) and repeat hospital stay (HR: 0.81; 95 % CI: 0.45–1.46) did not differ between the groups. The primary endpoint was significantly reduced in patients with elevated troponin on admission (HR: 0.43; 95 % CI: 0.23–0.80), but not in those with normal troponin (HR: 1.67; 95 % CI: 0.75–3.70; p for interaction=0.03) Table 6.2.

In this important study, the authors determined that these results do not allow a definite conclusion about the benefit of an EA approach when applied systematically among elderly patients with NSTEACS. The finding of a significant interaction of the treatment effect according to troponin status at baseline should be confirmed in a larger sized trial Fig. 6.5.

Based on these study results, the same group evaluated the cause of death within 1 year of hospital admission in patients with non-ST-segment elevation acute coronary syndromes in patients aged ≥75 years [31]. From January 2008 through May 2010, 645 patients were enrolled aged ≥75 years with non-ST-segment elevation acute coronary syndromes: 313 in a randomized trial comparing an early aggressive

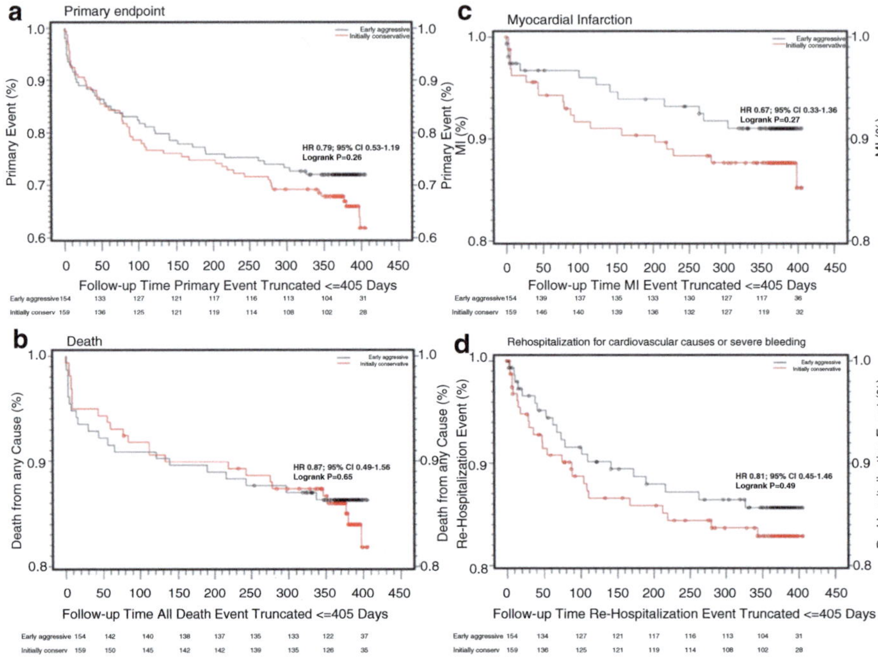

Fig. 6.5 Kaplan-Meier survival curves for the primary outcome early aggressive vs. initially conservative approach in elderly ACS-patients (**a–d**), all-cause mortality, MI and repeat hospital stay (Adapted from Ref. [30] with permission)

versus an initially conservative approach, and 332, excluded from the trial for specific reasons, in a parallel registry. Each death occurring during 1 year of follow-up, was adjudicated by an independent committee. The mean age was 82 years in both study cohorts and 53 % were men. By the end of the follow-up period (median 369 days, interquartile range 345–391), 120 patients (18.6 %) had died. The mortality was significantly greater in the registry (23.8 % vs 13.1 %, p=0.001). The deaths were classified as cardiac in 94 % of the cases during the index admission and 68 % of the cases during the follow-up period. Eighty-six percent of the cardiac deaths were of ischemic origin. In a multivariate logistic regression model, that included the variables present on admission in the whole study population, the ejection fraction (hazard ratio 0.95, 95 % confidence interval 0.94–0.97; p<0.001), hemoglobin level (hazard ratio 0.85, 95 % confidence interval 0.76–0.94; p=0.001), older age (hazard ratio 1.05, 95 % confidence interval 1.01–1.10, p=0.010) and creatinine clearance (hazard ratio 0.99, 95 % confidence interval 0.97–0.99; p=0.030) were the independent predictors of all-cause death at 1 year. The authors established that in this elderly patient group, within 1 year after admission for non-ST-segment elevation acute coronary syndromes, most deaths in patients aged ≥75 years have a cardiac origin, mostly as a result of myocardial ischemia.

It is unclear whether the benefits of an early invasive strategy (EIS) in patients with non-ST-segment elevation acute coronary syndromes (NSTEACS) equally applies to younger and older individuals, as elderly patients are generally less likely to undergo EIS when compared to younger patients. Consequently, the same group performed a meta-analysis, to compare the benefit of an EIS versus a selectively invasive strategy (SIS) in patients with NSTEACS, to test if the benefit of an EIS over a SIS applies to older individuals [32]. The authors extracted data from randomized controlled trials (RCTs), identified through search methodology filters. The primary outcome of the analysis was the composite of all-cause death and myocardial infarction (MI). Secondary outcomes were death and MI taken alone and re-hospitalization. Nine trials (n = 9400 patients) were eligible. The incidence of the composite end-point of MI and all-cause death was 16.0 % with the EIS and 18.3 % with the SIS (OR: 0.85, 95 % CI: 0.76–0.95). The incidence of MI was 8.4 % with the EIS and 10.9 % with the SIS (OR: 0.75, 95 % CI: 0.66–0.87). Similar results were obtained for re-hospitalization (OR: 0.71, 95 % CI: 0.55–0.90). The incidence of all-cause death did not differ between the two groups. However, the EIS reduced the composite end-point and re-hospitalization to a greater extent in elderly than in younger patients (P for interaction = 0.044 and <0.0001, respectively). These findings were confirmed in meta-regression analyses. The authors concluded, that in patients with NSTEACS, a routine EIS reduces the risk of re-hospitalization and the composite end point of recurrent MI and death, to a greater extent in elderly than in younger individuals.

Conclusion

In the light of the above mentioned data, older patients presenting with an acute coronary syndrome (ACS) in general have a broader spectrum of clinical presentation and higher complication rates when undergoing treatment, either interventionally or conservatively.

These patients should not be treated differently from younger patients, since they gain the greatest benefit from interventional treatment. However, more caution evaluating benefits and risks of usual therapies should be applied. The consideration of remaining life expectancy, quality of life and patient preferences and values is more important for clinical decision making than in younger patients. Future work has to be done:

- to identify the most efficient assessment tools that provides clinicians and patients with useful information for the kind of treatment and outcome after any treatment
- to determine and to identify patients and their preconditions (comorbidities and functional capacity), which should lead to intervention or deferral from interventional therapy and to the identification of patients, who benefit most from intervention
- to determine adequate outcome measurements after 6 months for both groups (death, myocardial infarction, stroke, frailty, functional capacity, pain relief) in

order to determine factors, which may be more effective and more suitable in the prediction of outcomes in NSTEMI in elderly patients (as it reveals functional, cognitive and behavioral deficits, which may play a decisive role)
- to evaluate patient wishes regarding the aim of the therapy in the presence of stable angina and acute coronary syndromes as well.

Furthermore advances in interventional skills, for instance the increasing use of the radial approach, development of adjunctive drug therapy and the increasing use of a multidisciplinary decision making process in these patients, will help to improve the results when treating elderly patients with ACS.

References

1. Gilat D, Goldbourt U, Reicher-Reiss H, Zion M, Kaplinksi E, Behar S. Prognosis of acute myocardial infarct in the elderly – SPRINT Study Group. Harefuah. 1993;124:601–3.
2. Alexander KP, Newby LK, Armstrong PW, Gibler WB, Rich MW, Van de Werf F, White HD, Weaver WD, Naylor MD, Gore JM, Krumholz HM, Ohman EM, American Heart Association Council on Clinical Cardiology, Society of Geriatric Cardiology. Acute coronary care in the elderly, part I. ST segment elevation myocardial infarction. Circulation. 2007;115:2549–69.
3. Alexander KP, Newby LK, Armstrong PW, Gibler WB, Rich MW, Van de Werf F, White HD, Weaver WD, Naylor MD, Gore JM, Krumholz HM, Ohman EM, American Heart Association Council on Clinical Cardiology, Society of Geriatric Cardiology. Acute coronary care in the elderly, part II. ST segment elevation myocardial infarction. Circulation. 2007;115:2570–89.
4. Fox KA, Anderson Jr FA, Dabbous OH, Steg PG, López-Sendón J, Van de Werf F, Budaj A, Gurfinkel EP, Goodman SG, Brieger D, GRACE investigators. Intervention in acute coronary syndromes: do patients undergo intervention on the basis of their risk characteristics? The Global Registry of Acute Coronary Events (GRACE). Heart. 2007;93:177–82.
5. Antman EM, Hand M, Armstrong PW, Bates ER, Green LA, Halasyamani LK, Hochman JS, Krumholz HM, Lamas GA, Mullany CJ, Pearle DL, Sloan MA, Smith SC Jr; 2004 Writing Committee Members, Anbe DT, Kushner FG, Ornato JP, Jacobs AK, Adams CD, Anderson JL, Buller CE, Creager MA, Ettinger SM, Halperin JL, Hunt SA, Lytle BW, Nishimura R, Page RL, Riegel B, Tarkington LG, Yancy CW. 2007 Focused Update of the ACC/AHA 2004 Guidelines for the Management of Patients With ST-Elevation Myocardial Infarction: a report of the American College of Cardiology/American Heart Association Task Force on Practice Guidelines: developed in collaboration with the Canadian Cardiovascular Society endorsed by the American Academy of Family Physicians: 2007 Writing Group to Review New Evidence and Update the ACC/AHA 2004 Guidelines for the Management of Patients With ST-Elevation Myocardial Infarction, Writing on Behalf of the 2004 Writing Committee. Circulation 2008;117:296–329.
6. Yusuf S, Flather M, Pogue J, Hunt D, Varigos J, Piegas L, Avezum A, Anderson J, Keltai M, Budaj A, Fox K, Ceremuzynski L. Variations between countries in invasive cardiac procedures and outcomes in patients with suspected unstable angina or myocardial infarction without initial ST-elevation. OASIS (Organisation to Assess Strategies for Ischaemic Syndromes) Registry Investigators. Lancet. 1998;352:507–14.
7. Granger CB, Goldberg RJ, Dabbous O, Pieper KS, Eagle KA, Cannon CP, Van De Werf F, Avezum A, Goodman SG, Flather MD, Fox KA, Global Registry of Acute Coronary Events Investigators. Predictors of hospital mortality in the global registry of acute coronary events. Arch Intern Med. 2003;163:2345–53.
8. Lee PY, Alexander KP, Hammill BG, Pasquali SK, Peterson ED. Representation of elderly persons and women in published randomized trials of acute coronary syndromes. JAMA. 2001;286:708–13.

9. Windecker S, for the TASK Force on Myocardial Revascularization of the European Society of Cardiology (ESC) and the European Association of Percutaneous Cardiovascular Interventions (EAPCI). 2014 ESC/EACTS Guidelines on myocardial revascularization. Eur Heart J. 2014;35:2541–619.
10. Bach RG, Cannon CP, Weintraub WS, DiBattiste PM, Demopoulos LA, Anderswon HV, DeLucca PT, Mahoney EM, Murphy SA, Braunwald E. The effect of routine, early invasive management on outcome for elderly patients with NSTEMI ACS. Ann Intern Med. 2004;141:186–95.
11. Avezum A, Makdisse M, Spencer F, Gore JM, Fox KA, Montalescot G, Eagle KA, White K, Mehta RH, Knobel E, Collet JE, Grace Investigators. Impact of age on management and outcome of ACS: observations from the GRACE registry. Am Heart J. 2005;149:67–73.
12. Mehta R, Rathore SS, Radford MJ, Wang Y, Wang Y, Krumholz HM. Acute myocardial infarction in the elderly: differences by age. J Am Coll Cardiol. 2001;38:736–41.
13. Vogt A, Bonzel T, Harmjanz D, von Leitner ER, Pfafferott C, Engel HJ, Niederer W, Schuster PR, Glunz HG, Neuhaus KL. PTCA registry of German community hospitals. Arbeitsgemeinschaft Leitender Kardiologischer Krankenhausärzte (ALKK) Study Group. Eur Heart J. 1997;18(7):1110–4.
14. De Servi S, Cavallini C, Dellavalle A, Santoro GM, Bonizzoni E, Marzocchi A, Politi A, Pesaresi A, Mariani M, Chierchia S, for the ROSAI-2 Investigators. Non-ST-elevation acute coronary syndrome in the elderly: Treatment strategies and 30-day outcome. Am Heart J. 2004;147:830–6.
15. Bahrmann P, Heppner HJ, Christ M, Bertsch T, Sieber CC. Early detection of non-ST-elevation myocardial infarction in geriatric patients by a new high-sensitive cardiac troponin T assay. Aging Clin Exp Res. 2012;24:290–4.
16. Christ M, Bertsch T, Popp S, Bahrmann P, Heppner HJ, Müller C. High-sensitivity troponin assays in the evaluation of patients with acute chest pain in the emergency department. Clin Chem Lab Med. 2011;49:1955–63.
17. Bahrmann P, Bahrmann A, Breithardt O-A, et al. Additional diagnostic and prognostic value of copeptin ultra-sensitive for diagnosis of non-ST-elevation myocardial infarction in older patients presenting to the emergency department. Clin Chem Lab Med. 2013;51:1307–19.
18. Bahrmann P, Christ M, Bahrmann A, et al. A 3-hour diagnostic algorithm for non-ST-elevation myocardial infarction using high sensitivity cardiac troponin T in unselected older patients presenting to the emergency department. J Am Med Dir Assoc. 2013;14:409–16.
19. Morrison DA, Bles RD, Sacks J. Coronary angioplasty for elderly patients with "high risk" unstable angina: short-term outcomes and long-term survival. J Am Coll Cardiol. 1997;143:339–44.
20. Devlin G, Gore JM, Elliott J, et al. GRACE Investigators. Management and 6-month outcomes in elderly and very elderly patients with high-risk non-ST-elevation acute coronary syndromes: The Global Registry of Acute Coronary Events. Eur Heart J. 2008;10:1275–82.
21. Rittger H, Schnupp S, Sinha A-M, et al. Predictors of treatment in acute coronary syndromes in the elderly. Catheter Cardiovasc Interv. 2012;80:735–43.
22. Morici N, De Servi S, Toso A, Murena E, Piscione F, Bolognese L, Petronio AS, Antonicelli R, Cavallini C, Angeli F, Savonitto S. Renal dysfunction, coronary revascularization and mortality among elderly patients with non ST elevation acute coronary syndrome. Eur Heart J Acute Cardiovasc Care. 2014. [Epub ahead of print].
23. Muñoz JC, Alonso JJ, Duran JM, Gimeno F, Ramos B, Garcimartin I, de la Fuente L, Gomez I, Fernandez-Aviles F. Coronary stent implantation in patients older than 75 years of age. Am Heart J. 2002;143:620–6.
24. Bauer T, Koeth O, Jünger C, Heer T, Wienbergen H, Gitt A, Zahn R, Senges J, Zeymer U; for the Acute Coronary Syndromes Registry (ACOS) et al. for the ACOS Investigators. Effect of an invasive strategy on in-hospital outcome on elderly patients with non-ST-elevation myocardial infarction. Eur Heart J. 2007;28:2873–8.
25. Rittger H, Hochadel M, Behrens S, Hauptmann KE, Zahn R, Mudra H, Brachmann J, Zeymer U. Interventional treatment and outcome in elderly patients with stable coronary artery disease. Results from the German ALKK registry. Herz. 2014;39:212–8.

26. Leontyev S, Walther T, Borger MA, Lehmann S, Finkat AK, Rastan A, Kempfert J, Falk V, Mohr FW. Aortic valve replacement in octogenarians: utility of risk stratification with EuroSCORE. Ann Thorac Surg. 2009;87:1440–5.
27. Schoenenberger AW, Radovanovic D, Stauffer JC. Age-related differences in the use of guideline-recommended medical and interventional therapie for acute coronary syndromes. A cohort study. J Am Geriatr Soc. 2008;56:510–6.
28. Schoenenberger AW, Stortecky S, Neumann S. Predictors of functional decline in elderly patients undergoing transcatheter aortic valve implantation (TAVI). Eur Heart J. 2013;34:684–92. doi:10.1093/eurheartj/ehs304.
29. Rittger H, Rieber J, Kögler K, Sinha AM, Schmidt M, Breithardt OA, Biggar P, Einsle F, Diegeler A, Brachmann J. Clinical outcome and quality of life after interventional treatment of left main disease with drug-eluting stents in comparison to CABG in elderly and younger patients. Clin Res Cardiol. 2011;100:439–46.
30. Savonitto S, Cavallini C, Petronio S, Murena E, Antonicelly R, Sacco A, Steffenino G, Bonechi F, Mossuti E, Manari A, Tolaro S, Toso A, Daniotti A, Piscione F, Morici N, Cesana B, Jori C, De Servi S. Early aggressive versus initially conservative treatment in elderly patients with non-ST-segment elevation acute coronary syndrome. J Am Coll Cardiol Cardiovasc Interv. 2012;5:906–16.
31. Morici N, Savonitto S, Murena E, Antonicelly R, Piovaccari G, Tucci D, Tamburino C, Fontanelli A, Bolognese L, Menozzi M, Cavallini C, Petronio AS, Ambrosio G, Piscione F, Steffenino G, De Servi S. Causes of death in patients ≥75 years of age with non-ST-segment elevation acute coronary syndrome. Am J Cardiol. 2013;112:1–7.
32. Angeli F, Verdeccia P, Savonitto S, Morici N, De Servi S, Vavallini C. Early invasive versusu selectively invasive strategy in patients with non-ST-segment elevation acute coronary syndrome: impact of age. Catheter Cardiovasc Interv. 2014;83:686–701.

Chapter 7
CABG Versus PCI in Elderly Patients

Harald Rittger

Introduction

Octogenarians represent an increasing proportion of patients admitted to hospital for revascularization due to coronary artery disease (CAD), either for percutaneous coronary intervention (PCI) or coronary artery bypass graft (CABG). This patient group is the fastest growing part of the population in the industrialized world with life expectancies being predicted to 77.1 years for men and 81.9 years for women in 2030 in the US [1]. This rapidly rising entity (including the top of the baby boomer generation), will crowd the "nursing homes" in about 30 years and consequently lead to a dramatic increase of patients with multivessel disease. About 40 % of people aged 80 years and more suffer from coronary heart disease which is accountable for >50 % of the mortality in this group [2].

In general there are three options to treat such patients: medical therapy, coronary intervention or surgery. Comorbidity and a lower physiological reserve distinguish this patient group substantially from younger patients, leading to consequences for the treatment options for elderly patients. Logically, in comparison to younger patients, worse outcomes are reported, with a higher morbidity and mortality for both – intervention and surgery. Moreover, effectiveness of different treatment regimens are still poorly evaluated due to the fact, that advanced age was an exclusion criteria in most of the studies [3, 4].

In fact, in everyday clinical practice elderly patients are often primarily directed to percutaneous interventions due to the assumption, that PCI offers a lower risk during the procedure, a risk that may even be too high for most of the octogenarians. In summary, both PCI and CABG offer advantages over medical therapy. PCI shows a lower in-hospital morbidity and mortality, while CABG-procedure in the long run,

H. Rittger, MD
Department of Internal Medicine I, Cardiology and Pneumology, Klinikum Fuerth, Fuerth, Germany
e-mail: harald.rittger@uk-erlangen.de

H. Rittger (ed.), *Interventional Cardiology in the Elderly*,
DOI 10.1007/978-3-319-21142-8_7

shows lower mortality and less reinterventions, however at the cost of a significantly higher stroke rate. When treating elderly patients, one of the main question remains, how relevant long term outcome in patients beyond 85 years is – a questions that up to now has not been answered. Furthermore, there is currently no data available concerning patient anticipations and wishes after coronary intervention and CABG procedure. Therefore, the main challenge for physicians in this context is, how to advise elderly patients: which of the treatment alternatives are best suited for an individual patient. This task can be considered difficult in the light of at least partially conflicting or non present evidence in the treatment of elderly patients with CAD Table 7.1.

Differences to a Younger Patient Cohort

According to recent ESC guidelines for myocardial revascularization in younger patient cohorts, angina is associated with the following: reduced exercise capacity, reduced quality of life, mental depression and repeated hospitalizations [5]. This is where the disparity to an elderly population becomes apparent. Elderly patients will probably not experience ischemia as angina, which will become noticeable as a decline in exercise capacity, congestive heart failure, dyspnea or, in some cases even as confusion or delirium. Albeit the incidence of CAD is growing with advanced age, with autopsy studies suggesting a prevalence of at least 70 % in patients >70 years, however only 15–30 % of the patients over 65 years show clinical signs of CAD. The discrepancy between clinical and autopsy prevalence implicates, that CAD often is silent and goes undetected in this patient group. This is underlined by a significantly reduced angina detection in elderly patients. Rittger et al. showed in a study of 101 patients undergoing PCI, in repeated balloon inflations during PCI, a significantly reduced pain sensitivity in patients >69 years compared with a younger patient group [6]. Another study by Ambepitiya et al. [7], investigated age-associated changes in pain perception, by comparing the time delay between the onset of ST-segment depression and the onset of AP during exercise stress testing. The authors found a significant difference of the mean delay to onset of pain, which was 49 s in patients aged 70–82 years and 30s in patients aged 42–59 years. One can conclude from these results, that there is an age dependent reduction in pain sensitivity, independent of objective signs of ischemia and of ischemic preconditioning. The reasons for the diminished pain perception in the elderly patient cohort remain unclear. Ambepitiya et al. postulated that peripheral mechanisms such as changes in the myocardial autonomic nerve endings with blunted ischemic pain perception, as well as changes in central nervous mechanisms, may be a cause for this phenomenon. Another theory suggested, that the higher prevalence of silent myocardial ischemia and infarction in elderly patients with CAD may be related to increased levels of endogenous opioids and increased opioid receptor sensitivity [8]. This explanation does not appear likely, as studies have demonstrated a similar increase in response of beta-endorphin levels to exercise in both elderly and younger patients [9].

Table 7.1 Effect of different revascularization strategies vs. medical treatment on angina, exercise time and number of medications in an overall population

Study	Angina		Exercise time		Number of medications	
	Early	Late	Early	Late	Early	Late
ACME	64 % vs. 46 %* free of angina at 6 months	62 % vs. 47 %* free of angina at 3 years	11.2 min vs. 9.5* min exercise time duration at 6 months	10.0 min vs. 8.5* min exercise time duration at 3 years	30 % vs. 50 % on ß-blocker*, 35 % vs. 71 % on CCB*, and 24 % vs. 50 % on nitrate* at 6 months	28 % vs. 39 % on ß-blocker, 47 % vs. 72 % on CCB*, and 24 % vs. 52 % on nitrate* at 3 years
RITA-2	19.4 % vs. 35.9 %* at 3 months	15.0 % vs. 21.4 %* at 5 years	37 s in favor of PCI* at 3 months	25 s in favor of PCI* at 3 years	37 % vs. 57 % on ≥2 drugs at 3 months	31 % vs. 45 % on ≥2 drugs at 5 years
AVERT	Improvement in angina 54 % vs. 41 %* at 1.5 years	–	–	–	61 % vs. 60 % on ß-blocker, 44 % vs. 49 % on CCB, and 50 % vs. 60 % on nitrate at 1.5 years	–
TIME	Significant improvement in angina class at 6 months	No differences in angina class at 1 year	–	–	Significant reduction of number of drugs at 6 months	Significant reduction of number of drugs at 1 year
MASS II	21 % (PCI) vs. 12 % (CABG) vs. 54 % (MT) free of angina* at 1 year	41 % (PCI) vs. 36 % (CABG) vs. 57 % (MT) free of angina* at 10 years	–	–	–	–

(continued)

Table 7.1 (continued)

Study	Angina		Exercise time		Number of medications	
	Early	Late	Early	Late	Early	Late
SWISSI II	–	–	Max workload at bicycle ergometry 169 W vs. I48 W* at 4 years	Max workload at bicycle ergometry I73 W vs. 136 W* at 10 years	49 % vs. 86 % on ß-blocker*,21 % vs. 51 % on CCB*, and 12 % vs. 47 % on nitrate* at 4 years	39 % vs. 84 % on ß-blocker*, 17 % vs. 32 % on CCB, and 4 % vs. 45 % on nitrate* at 10 years
COURAGE	56 % vs. 47 %* free of angina at 6 months	59 % vs. 56 % free of angina at 3 years	–	–	85 % vs. 89 % on ß-blocker, 40 % vs. 49 % on CCB*, and 53 % vs. 67 % on nitrate* at 1 year	85 % vs. 86 % on ß-blocker, 42 % vs. 52 % on CCB*, and 40 % vs. 57 % on nitrate* at 5 years

ESC guidelines on myocardial revascularization 2014; adapted from Ref. [5] with permission
*P<0.05

CCB calcium-channel blocker, *PCI* percutaneous coronary intervention, *CABG* coronary artery bypass grafting, *MT* medical therapy, *W* watts

Additionally, animal studies show a decrease in opioid receptor responsiveness with advancing age [10].

Moreover, with advanced age, it will become more difficult to perform ischemia testing in suspected CAD, since many elderly patients will not be able to carry out exercise tests due to physical disabilities (e.g. degenerative joint disease). Consequently, the detection of CAD in elderly patients prior to any diagnostic or therapeutic intervention, appears to be difficult in light of other age specific changes.

Results for PCI in Multivessel Disease

The success of CABG-surgery in earlier days has been attributed to the greater efficacy of surgery to achieve a complete revascularization in the setting of multivessel- and left main disease. Nevertheless, in the growing elderly population there are plenty of reasons to justify the search for alternatives to surgery. Many of these patients will have a higher risk for perioperative complications: for instance myocardial infarction, prolonged mechanical ventilation, pneumonia and especially neurological events. For a high percentage, the indication to perform CABG procedure with an even higher postoperative morbidity rate, seems at least to be questionable. Especially in view of the presumably preferred outcomes in the elderly, (since there is no data available about patients anticipations to revascularization) – namely to maintain their functional status and quality of life. The search for alternatives to CABG therefore has partially liberated the evolution of interventional cardiology.

There are plenty of trials evaluating the effectiveness of angioplasty in the treatment of multivessel disease, prior to the era of stenting and the introduction of DES in interventional cardiology. However, it is interesting to point out, that contrary to the present evidence in coronary bypass grafting, besides the TIME-trial (which compared the effect of coronary intervention with stenting in comparison to medical treatment alone), currently no randomized trial exists, which was exclusively performed in an elderly population. The majority of all trials were performed in an overall population, with subgroup analyses for elderly patients in some trials and the vast majority of the present evidence comes from retrospective analyses.

Starting with the balloon era in an overall population, the BARI-trial (Bypass Angioplasty Revascularization Investigation) as a milestone trial, showed an equivalent mortality rate after 30 days at the cost of a higher revascularization rate in patients receiving PCI (52 % vs. 6 % with CABG after 5 years) and a higher stroke rate in patients treated with CABG. However, it indicated a 5-year cardiac mortality in patients with multivessel disease, which was significantly greater after initial treatment with PTCA than with CABG. The difference was manifest in diabetic patients on drug therapy: there were no significant differences overall for the composite end point of cardiac mortality or MI between treatment groups or for cardiac

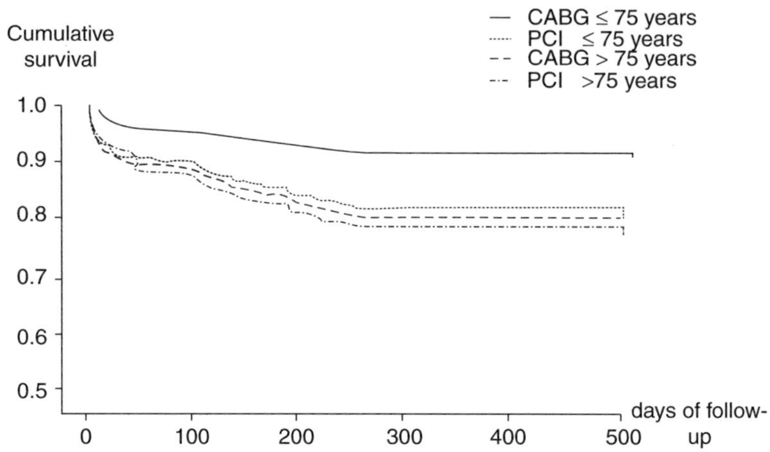

Fig. 7.1 Adjusted overall MACE rates at the end of follow-up, according to age and procedure (Adapted from Ref. [13] with permission)

mortality in nondiabetic patients, regardless of symptoms, left ventricular function, number of diseased vessels or stenotic proximal left anterior descending artery (Figs. 7.1 and 7.2) [11].

In the following decade, the implementation of stent techniques and the introduction of modern antiplatelet therapies has expanded the potential of interventional therapies substantially.

In the Alberta Provincial Project for outcomes Assessment in Coronary Heart Disease (APPROACH) study, a large cohort of patients >70 years undergoing PCI were studied and their survival examined by prescribed treatment (CABG, PCI, or medical therapy) for patients in three age categories: <70 years, 70–79 years, and ≥80 years of age. In 15 392 patients, 4-year adjusted actuarial survival rates for CABG, PCI and medical therapy were 95.0 %, 93.8 %, and 90.5 %, respectively. In 5198 patients 70–79 years of age, survival rates were 87.3 %, 83.9 %, and 79.1 %, respectively. In 983 patients ≥80 years of age, survival was 77.4 % for CABG, 71.6 % for PCI, and 60.3 % for medical therapy. Absolute risk differences in comparison to medical therapy for CABG (17.0 %) and PCI (11.3 %) were greater for patients ≥80 years of age than for younger patients. After 4 years, those patients over 80 years had the poorest survival rate with medical therapy 60.3 %, PCI 71.6 % and CABG 77.4 %. In this study, for the first time, the so-called risk-paradoxon was described: elderly patients paradoxically had greater absolute risk reductions, associated with surgical or percutaneous revascularization, than do younger patients. The combination of these results with a recent randomized trial suggests, that the benefits of aggressive revascularization therapies may extend to subsets of patients in older age groups [12].

Nonetheless, one has to keep in mind that due to a lack of randomized data, that probably the fittest were chosen to receive surgery and those patients in a worse condition were given medical therapy.

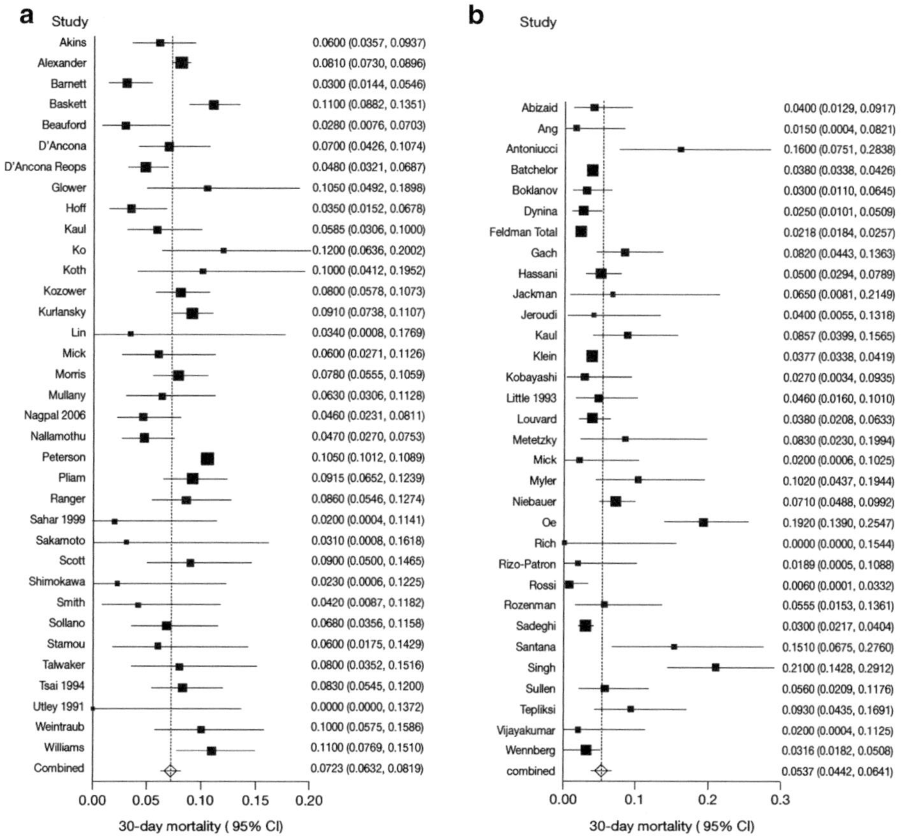

Fig. 7.2 Thirty day mortality rates for CABG (panel **a**) and PCI (panel **b**) in different studies (Adapted from Ref. [21] with permission)

Comparing the outcome of older versus younger patients with CABG-procedure in a series of 300 patients with left main disease, Rittger et al. showed, that there was no difference in outcome and quality of life between older and younger patients treated with PCI [13].

In the ARTS-trial, which randomized 600 patients to PCI and 605 patients to CABG, patients treated with surgery showed longer symptom free survival [14]. Despite having more complex lesions, results from stenting were better than in the BARI trial. Interestingly, advanced age was an independent predictor of unfavorable outcome in the CABG-, but not in the PCI group.

All other trials from this era, like the ERACI-2 trial, demonstrated a favorable 18-month mortality rate in the PCI group, however a higher reintervention rate [15]. The SOS-trial showed the same results, namely higher reintervention rates and lower stroke rates with PCI. It is interesting to note, that after 1 year in the SOS trial, quality of life and physical health status was comparable between the two groups in the elderly subgroups [16]. The only study with a predominantly elderly population was the AWESOME-study (more than 50 % of the patients enrolled were >67 years), which randomized patients with a high risk profile for cardiac shock or reduced LV-EF [17]. Results showed a similar outcome after 3 years regarding longterm mortality and quality of life.

The most recent SYNTAX-trial randomized patients with either left main or three-vessel disease to CABG or PCI, contrary to previous trials where patients received drug evading stents [18]. After 3 years there was no significant difference in the composite endpoint death, MI and stroke, with a higher rate of revascularization in the PCI group. Moreover, in this study the SYNTAX-Score was introduced, as an anatomical and morphologic grading tool in order to encompass the complexity of coronary artery disease. It consists of different angiographic scoring systems for the evaluation of bifurcations, the extent of calcifications and the presence of chronic occlusions. With a cut-off value of 33, it differentiates patients who will likely benefit from an intervention and those who will not, nota bene patients throughout all age groups. This score does include angiographic items and is able to predict reintervention rates, however not clinical outcomes of patients with multivessel disease. Furthermore, it is very helpful in the decision making process concerning the usefulness of coronary intervention or transferring to bypass surgery.

Again it is noteworthy, that all these trials have not been performed in an exclusively elderly population, which underlines the need for a randomized study in the elderly population.

Results for CABG

As already mentioned, all studies comparing different treatment strategies in the elderly, patients treated with PCI have a favorable short term outcome, however longterm outcome appears to be in favor of surgery. Compared to a younger population, in-hospital mortality rates for patients operated with stable coronary artery disease are higher than in younger patients and results are reported to be in a range between 2.2 and 9.7 %. Nevertheless, with the evolution of surgical techniques (e.g. off-cap-technique or the frequent use of the internal mammary artery), a significant and continuing drop in complication rates has been documented.

In an early study, CABG procedure in elderly patients was associated with a mortality rate of 24 % [20] and in comparison to a recent meta-analysis of 65 studies juxtaposing CABG surgery with PCI, reported a 30 day mortality of 5.3 % [21]. Since several studies confirm the decline in mortality rates [19, 22, 23], one could conclude, that age is not a prognostic parameter any longer, nonetheless age is an incremental part of the two most predominantly used clinical scores, the STS and Euro-Score.

In a sequential cross sectional analysis in a single center retrospective study, examining 1062 consecutive patients 80 years and older with a mean age of 83 ± 2.8 years, Kurlansky and co found an in-hospital mortality of initially 9.7 %, which decreased to 2.2 % in the course of the study between 1989 and 2001.

In-hospital complications were reported at a rate of 33 % ranging from complications such as reoperation due to bleeding (3.2 %), perioperative myocardial infarction in 1.5 %, low cardiac output in 16.2 %, cardiac arrest 7.8 %, renal insufficiency in 9.8 %, respiratory insufficiency in 17.8 %, cerebrovascular accident 3.2 % and deep sternal infection in 1.5 %. The following independent correlations of hospital mortality were identified: date of surgery, arrhythmia, abnormal ejection fraction, renal insufficiency, non-elective surgery conduit type and reperfusion time.

Using Medicare claims data (with 10,141 patients with ACS and aged 85 years or older), Sheridan et al. discovered after 3 years early benefits, with lesser morbidity and mortality with PCI, however CABG outcomes improved by 3 years [24]. After 3 years 66 % patients receiving CABG survived, compared to 62.7 % of PCI recipients. 46.1 % of CABG patients were free from the composite endpoint (death, repeat revascularization, stroke, acute myocardial infarction) vs. 38.7 % of PCI patients. The authors concluded, that in very elderly patients with ACS, the operative treatment has advantages compared to PCI. Nevertheless, for optimization of these outcomes, patient selection requires the absence of the following: significant congestive heart failure, lung disease and peripheral vascular disease. According to Sheridan et al, after 3 years 60 % of patients of either treatment and after 5 years 50 % of patients >80 years are still alive.

This development can be attributed to the overall advanced operative skills of cardiac surgeons, for example the increasing use of the left internal mammarial artery. However, there is still no pattern, which can discriminate mortality in the elderly from a younger population and despite all advances in cardiac surgery, stroke rate remains twice as high in the elderly patient group [21, 25].

Interestingly, contrary to the observed mortality drop, morbidity does not decrease. In a population, which is getting older and older, with an increased comorbid burden, one can imagine, that mortality is hence not the sole and the adequate parameter of operative outcome. Retrieval of functional status, the ability to perform activities of daily life when returning to the own home, are goals which are perhaps more warranted by the elderly population than absolute gain in life years.

CABG Versus PCI

As outlined before, randomized studies as well as large registries have demonstrated, that for intervention as well as for surgery, better outcomes and an improved quality of life compared to medical treatment. Nonetheless, it is still unknown, which of the two treatment options performs better especially in elderly patients. Mc Kellar et al. reported in a meta-analysis of 66 studies comparing PCI vs. CABG in octogenarians, a pooled estimate of a 30 day mortality for the CABG group of 7.2 % (6.3–8.2 %) compared to 5.4 % (4.4–6.4 %) for the PCI group. One year survival was reported to be in a range of 86 % in the CABG vs. 87 % in the PCI group, 3 years survival was 78 % for both groups and 5-year survival was 68 % for the CABG- and 62 % for the PCI group [21] Table 7.2.

Table 7.2 Pooled estimates for short and long-term survival rates in patients treated with intervention or CABG-procedure

CABG and PCI studies	Pooled estimate	95 % CI
30 day mortality	6.3 %	5.3–7.4
1 year survival	86 %	84–88
3 year survival	78 %	74–81
5 year survival	67 %	61–72
CABG studies		
30 day mortality	7.2 %	6.3–8.2
1 year survival	86 %	83–88
3 year survival	78 %	74–82
5 year survival	68 %	62–73
PCI studies		
30 day mortality	5.4 %	4.4–6.4
1 year survival	87 %	84–91
3 year survival	78 %	68–87
5 year survival	62 %	46–77

Adapted from Ref. [21]
Abbreviations: *PCI* percutaneous coronary intervention

Table 7.3 Predictors of 30 day mortality rates

Variable	Estimate	*P* value
Predictor		
CABG	5.8 %	<0.001
Male gender	0.3 %	<0.001
Multivessel disease	0.07 %	0.001
Abnormal left ventricular ejection fraction	0.1 %	0.001
Protective		
More recent study	0.5 %	<0.001
Nonelective revascularization	0.04 %	0.02
Diabetes mellitus	0.3 %	<0.001

Adapted from Ref. [21]

The authors came to the conclusion, that revascularization can be performed in octogenarians with acceptable short-term and long-term outcomes; however, most of the evidence is, low level. Furthermore, it is unclear whether octogenarians derive a greater survival benefit from CABG or from PCI, as preprocedural risk profiles differ between intervention types. Periprocedural and long-term outcomes are nevertheless equivalent, therefor randomized, controlled trials of high-risk octogenarians are needed (Table 7.3).

Due to the lack of randomized studies the quality of available evidence is low level for octogenarians undergoing revascularization. This is impressively reflected in the review of McKellar, with 5 studies to compare 3 years survival and 3 studies to compare 5 years survival in this very elderly patient group. One reason for the lack of randomized studies could be, that physicians and patients are unwilling to randomize or participate in a study comparing PCI with CABG, since there is a common fear not to survive any of these alternatives, esp. the surgical one.

As the proportion of elderly patients increases, possibilities to perform a randomized study should increase. This study should incrementally include questions such as: quality of life, the regaining of functional status, neurological outcomes and should try to answer the main question of meaningful endpoints for elderly patients.

Selection Criteria

A major problem arising with retrospective analysis is the imminent selection bias for physicians and in part for the elderly patient itself, as only patients with an apparent low risk with surgery were included. For instance, those patients may have had less comorbid conditions and biological age may be less than expected, rehabilitation time may be shorter, et cetera.

Quantification of risk is problematic, since the STS-score as well as the new EuroScore II include age as one of the main risk factors for a higher operational risk Table 7.4.

To date there are no selection criteria known to differentiate between elderly patients whether it is preferable to operate or to intervene. The favorable and better short term outcomes in patients receiving PCI might put across, that PCI is the only alternative for those patients. However, as previously mentioned, the favorable long term outcomes for surgery, even for elderly and very elderly patients arises as a viable alternative to PCI.

But, again the question materializes whom to intervene and whom to operate? Following relative contraindications should be considered: poor left ventricular function with huge ischemic or scar territories, small vessels as bad anatomical target and diffuse disease of the coronaries including poor anatomical targets, lack of conduits which could serve as bypass grafts, reduced pulmonary function, anatomic conditions which prevent successful surgery like a porcelain aorta, bleeding, severe reduced life expectancy, metastatic cancer, liver dysfunction, advanced age >90 years and poor physical status including excessive frailty. Dealing with elderly patients the question arises, where does poor physical status begin? Is it a patient who is wheel chair bound and/or suffering from dementia and to which degree. We know very well it is not only mortality, that is important for elderly patients. The question emerges, if long term outcome really does play a major role in octogenarians. Are not other factors such as the prevention of functional decline, improvement in quality of life and ability to perform activities of daily life a more powerful goal? Therefore elderly patients should be given the choice between surgery, PCI and/or medical management. In an elderly population with multiple comorbidities, these issues are far more compelling than long term survival. Up to date there is no evidence, which expectations elderly patients have to any interventions, is it long-term outcome or improvement of the functional status?

Recent data suggest, that the use of frailty scores, gait speed and the estimate of functional status, provide better information for the assessment of perioperative risk [26, 27].

Table 7.4 Comparison of different studies using the Euroscore, Euroscore II and the STS-score to predict outcomes after revascularization

Author	No of patients	Inclusion	Design	Coronary procedures	Discrimination (c-statistic)			Calibration [goodness-of-fit (Hosmer-Lemershow)]		
					Log ES	ES II	STS	Log ES	ES II	STS
Biancari	1027	2006–2011	Retrospective, single-centre	(i)CABG	0.838	0.852	–	–	–	–
Kirmani	14,432	2001–2010	Retrospective, single-centre	66 % (i)CABG, 12 % CABG+valve	–	0.818	0.805	–	<0.001	<0.001
Kune	428	2004–2012	Retrospective, single-centre	(i)CABG	0.70	0.72	0.62	–	<0.01	0.10
Splliopoulos	216	1999–2005	Retrospective, single-centre	CABG+AVR	0.75	0.77	–	–	–	–
Wang	818	2010–2012	Retrospective, single-centre	(i)CABG	0.675	0.642	0.641	0.061 ($X^2=13.5$)	0.15 ($X^2=12.0$)	0.243 ($X^2=10.3$)
Chalmers	2913	2006–2010	Retrospective, single-centre	(i)CABG	0.77	0.79	–	0.41	0.052	–
Chalmers	517	2006–2010	Retrospective, single-centre	CABG+AVR	0.67	0.74	–	0.38	0.38	–
Carnero-Alcázar	1231	2005–2010	Retrospective, single-centre	(i)CABG	0.884	0.90	–	0.01 ($X^2=20.1$)	0.001 ($X^2=26.6$)	–
Carnero-Alcázar	301	2005–2010	Retrospective, single-centre	CABG+valve	0.779	0.827	–	0.029 ($X^2=17.3$)	0.334 ($X^2=9.1$)	–
Osnabrugge	16,096	2003–2012	Retrospective, multicenter	(i)CABG	–	0.77	0.81	–	STS score better in figure, no formal test	
Osnabrugge	1627	2003–2012	Retrospective, multicenter	CABG+AVR	–	0.74	0.76	–	–	–

Adapted from Ref. [5]

AVR aortic valve replacement, *CABG* coronary artery bypass graft, *(i)CABG* (isolated) coronary artery bypass grafting, *ES* EuroSCORE, *TS* Society of Thoracic Surgeons

In this regard it seems essential to inaugurate a new risk score exclusively made for elderly patients, which incorporates morphologic, clinical, as well as functional items like frailty, functional status and pre-existing quality of life.

Summary

How to deal with an aging population whilst facing increasing health care costs and decreasing resources for an optimal health care management, will be the decisive question in the upcoming years. Prospective trials and registries have shown comparable survival rates and increased quality of life, for patients treated with intervention or surgery [19, 21–23, 28]. Subsequently, overall invasive procedures, either PCI or CABG-procedure, show advantages over medical therapy. Among older adults both options increasingly provide better results regarding short term mortality and especially longterm mortality. Very elderly patients often suffer from poor functional status, cognitive impairment and plenty of comorbid conditions like chronic obstructive pulmonary disease, renal insufficiency and neurological disorders. Those patients definitely need an individualized management. The decision making process between invasive and medical treatment, can never be evidence-based, since randomized studies are lacking and hence it often appears to be virtually impossible. In summary all three options, medical management, intervention and surgery are viable options to treat an elderly patient with multitvessel disease. Which of these alternatives will be the most appropriate one for an individual patient, remains the most challenging question in this context: what are the main selection criteria for any therapy, is there an increased risk for any of these options, does the improvement in symptom relief and functional capacity justify the increased risk for complications, how sustainable is this improvement, what is wanted from the elderly population itself, what are the expectations of elderly patients, and finally is quality of life, is frailty or improvement in functional status the goal which should be reached?

References

1. US Census Bureau "2008 National Population Projections" released August 2008; www.census.gov/population/www/projections/2008projections.html.
2. National center for health statistics. National health interview survey 1983–1985. Hyattsville: The Center; 1986.
3. Gurwitz JH, Col NF, Avorn J. The exclusion of the elderly and women from clinical trials in acute myocardial infarction. JAMA. 1992;268:1417–22.
4. Lee PY, Alexander KP, Hammill BG, Pasquali SK, Peterson ED. Representation of elderly persons and women in published randomized trials of acute coronary syndromes. JAMA. 2001;286:708–13.
5. Windecker S, for the TASK Force on Myocardial Revascularization of the European Society of Cardiology (ESC) and the European Association of Percutaneous Cardiovascular Interventions (EAPCI). 2014 ESC/EACTS Guidelines on myocardial revascularization. Eur Heart J. 2014;35:2541–619.

6. Rittger H, Rieber J, Breithardt OA, Dücker M, Schmidt M, Abbara S, Sinha AM, Jakob A, Nölker G, Brachmann J. Influence of age on pain perception in acute myocardial ischemia: a possible cause for delayed treatment in older patients. Int J Cardiol. 2011;149:63–7.
7. Ambepitiyja G, Roberts M, Ranjadayalan K, Tallis R. Silent exertional myocardial ischemia in the elderly. A quantitative analysis of angina perceptual threshold and the influence of autonomic function. J Am Geriatr Soc. 1994;42:732–7.
8. Ellestadt MH, Kaun P. Naloxone and asymptomatic ischemia: failure to induce angina during exercise testing. Am J Cardiol. 1984;54:982–4.
9. Hatfield BD, Goldfarb AH, Sforzo GA, Flynn MG. Serum beta-endorphin and affective response to graded exercise in young and elderly men. J Gerontol. 1987;42:429–31.
10. Morley JE. Neuropeptides: behaviour and aging. J Am Geriatr Soc. 1986;34:52–61.
11. Chaitman BR, Rosen AD, Williams DO, et al. Myocardial infarction and cardiac mortality in the Bypass angioplasty revascularization investigation (BARI) randomized trial. Circulation. 1997;96:2162–70.
12. Graham MM, Ghali A, Faris P, et al. Survival after coronary revascularization in the elderly. Circulation. 2002;105:2378–84.
13. Rittger H, Rieber J, Kögler K, Sinha AM, Schmidt M, Breithardt OA, Biggar P, Einsle F, Diegeler A, Brachmann J. Clinical outcome and quality of life after interventional treatment of left main disease with drug-eluting stents in comparison to CABG in elderly and younger patients. Clin Res Cardiol. 2011;100:439–46.
14. Serruys PW, Ong ATL, Herwerden LA, et al. Five-year outcomes after coronary stenting versus bypass surgery for the treatment of multivessel disease – the final analysis of the arterial revascularization therapy study (ARTS) randomized trial. J Am Coll Cardiol. 2005;46:575–81.
15. Rodriguez AR, Baldi J, Pereira CF, Navia J, Alemparte MR, Delacasa A, Vigo F, Vogel D, O'Neill W, Palacios I. Five-year follow-up of the argentine randomized trial of coronary angioplasty with stenting versus coronary bypass surgery in patients with multiple vessel disease (ERACI II). J Am Coll Cardiol. 2005;46:582–8.
16. Zhang Z, Mahoney EM, Spertus JA, et al. The impact of age on outcomes after coronary artery bypass surgery versus stent-assisted percutaneous coronary intervention: one-year results from the Stent or Surgery (SoS) trial. Am Heart J. 2006;152:1153–60.
17. Morrison DA, Sethi G, Sacks J, et al. Percutaneous coronary intervention versus coronary artery bypass graft surgery for patients with medically refractory myocardial ischemia and risk factors for adverse outcomes with bypass: a multicenter, randomized trial. Investigators of the Department of Veterans Affairs Cooperative Study Number 385, the Angina with Extremely Serious Operative Mortality Evaluation (AWESOME). J Am Coll Cardiol. 2001;38:143–9.
18. Kappetein AP, Feldmann TE, Mack MJ, Morice MC, Holmes DR, Stahle E, Dawkins KD, Mohr FW, Serruys PW, Colombo A. Comparison of coronary bypass surgery with drug-eluting stenting for the treatment of left main and/or three-vessel disease: three year follow up of the SYNTAX trial. Eur Heart J. 2011;32:2125–34.
19. Kurlansky PA, Williams DB, Traad EA, Zucker M, Ebra G. Eighteen-year follow-up demonstrates prolonged survival and enhanced quality of life for octogenarians after coronary artery bypass grafting. J Thorac Cardiovasc Surg. 2011;141:394–9.
20. Edmunds LH, Stephenson LW, Edie RN, Ratcliffe MB. Open-heart surgery in octogenarians. N Engl J Med. 1988;318:131–6.
21. Mc Kellar SH, Brown ML, Frye RL, Schaff HV, Sundt III TM. Comparison of coronary revascularization procedures in octogenarians: a systematic review and meta-analysis. Nat Clin Pract Cardiovasc Med. 2008;5:738–46.
22. Saxena A, Dinh DT, Yap CH, et al. Critical analysis of early and late outcomes after isolated coronary artery bypass surgery in elderly patients. Ann Thorac Surg. 2011;92:1702–11.
23. Li Z, Amsterdam EA, Yeo KK, et al. Coronary artery bypass operations for elderly patients in California, 2003 to 2008. Ann Thorac Surg. 2012;93:1167–73.
24. Sheridan BC, Stearns SC, Rossi JS, D'Arcy LP, Federspiel JJ, Carey TS. Three-year outcomes of multivessel revascularization in very elderly acute coronary syndrome patients. Ann Thorac Surg. 2010;89:1889–95.

25. Alexander KP, Anstrom KJ, Mühlbaier LH, et al. Outcomes of cardiac surgery in patients age >80 ys: results from the National Cardiovascular Network. J Am Coll Cardiol. 2000;35: 731–8.
26. Afilalo J, Eisenberg MJ, Morin JF, et al. Gait speed as an incremental predictor of mortality and major morbidity in elderly patients undergoing cardiac surgery. J Am Coll Cardiol. 2010;56:1668–76.
27. Afilalo J, Mottillo B, Eisenberg MJ, et al. Addition of frailty and disability to cardiac surgical risk scores identifying elderly patients at high risk of mortality and major morbidity. Circ Cardiovasc Qual Outcomes. 2013;5:222–8.
28. The TIME Investigators. Trial of invasive versus medical therapy in elderly patients with chronic symptomatic coronary-artery disease (TIME): a randomized trial. Lancet. 2001;358: 951–7.

Chapter 8
Non-coronary Interventions in the Elderly

Ralf Birkemeyer

Introduction

Surgical repair has been the predominant curative approach to valvular heart disease in the industrialized nations during the last decade in spite of the fact that mitral valvuloplasty is the usual approach to rheumatic mitral stenosis with fused commissures. Rheumatic valve disease, however, has fairly declined due to the decrease of rheumatic fever. Degenerative aetiology of valvular disease especially of the aortic valve is now predominant and prevails in the elderly population [1–3].

As surgical risk is largely dependent on age and age-related comorbidities [4, 5] a substantial proportion of affected patients are deemed no appropriate candidates for open heart surgery.

The European Heart Survey from 2001 showed that about 30 % of patients aged >75 years with severe aortic stenosis and an accepted indication for aortic valve replacement were managed conservatively. In patients with severe, symptomatic mitral regurgitation of predominantly degenerative and ischemic aetiologies only 49 % had a surgical repair. In both cohorts age was the main extra-cardiac reason for non-surgical treatment [1, 6].

Although prognostic considerations might be a minor issue for the very elderly with valve disease the symptomatic limitation of daily activities or even symptoms at rest can have detrimental effects on quality of life in patients with prohibitive or high surgical risk [7, 8]. An interventional repair of the underlying structural problem avoiding the trauma of open heart surgery has been considered an interesting alternative in this patient subset for quite a while. Balloon aortic valvuloplasty for aortic stenosis in the elderly was established in 1986. In spite of good initial hemodynamic improvement mid-term results after a few months were rather disappoint-

R. Birkemeyer, MD
Interventional Cardiology, Herzklinik Ulm, Ulm, Germany
e-mail: ralf.birkemeyer@herzklinik-ulm.de

H. Rittger (ed.), *Interventional Cardiology in the Elderly*,
DOI 10.1007/978-3-319-21142-8_8

ing [9, 10]. Only recently new interventional technologies like transcatheter aortic valve replacement for aortic stenosis and transcatheter repair for mitral insufficiency have been introduced as appropriate options for causal long-term treatment in non-surgical patients [11, 12].

In addition transcatheter mitral repair has emerged as supplementary therapy in heart failure patients with functional mitral insufficiency. Surgical repair in this cohort of patients is not generally recommended due to equivocal study results [13].

Another emerging non-coronary intervention without established surgical alternative is left atrial appendage closure in patients with atrial fibrillation and contraindication for long term anticoagulation [14, 15]. Both conditions are predominantly encountered in the elderly due to the increasing prevalence of coronary artery disease and atrial fibrillation with age [16, 17]. Furthermore age is an important determinant of bleeding risk [18].

Interventional closure has also been established for different types of shunts like in atrial septal defects. Detecting significant atrial septal defects in elderly patients raises rather the question of closing the defect at all than how to close.

Paravalvular leaks after surgical valve replacement and post-myocardial infarction ventricular septal defects are rare causes of significant shunts or hemolysis. They might however require urgent treatment. Preference of a surgical or interventional approach is a highly individualized decision with the lack of general recommendations.

Balloon Aortic Valvuloplasty and Transcatheter Aortic Valve Replacement

Degenerative aortic stenosis is a typical disease of the elderly population (>70 years) with frequent denial of surgery due to a prohibitive or high surgical risk [19, 20]. Degenerative disease can manifest earlier with additional valve pathology (bicuspid valve or rheumatic disease). Once symptoms have occurred spontaneous prognosis is poor with the majority of patients being dead within 5 years after onset of angina, 3 years after syncope and 2 years after onset of heart failure [21, 22].

Balloon aortic valvuloplasty (BAV) was introduced for symptomatic relief in non-surgical patients in 1986 [23]. Initial hemodynamic improvement after stand-alone valvuloplasty was however of short duration due to early recoil of the stretched aortic annulus and further leaflet calcification. At that time the BAV procedure also had a rather high complication rate (e.g. vascular injury, ventricular perforation, massive aortic regurgitation, annulus rupture, embolic events) which has been overcome with further advancement of technique and materials [24]. Due to these limitations the method had been largely abandoned by the 1990s. In the era of transcatheter aortic valve replacement aortic valvuloplasty has been incorporated in the procedure. Stand-alone valvuloplasty might still be an option in some multi-

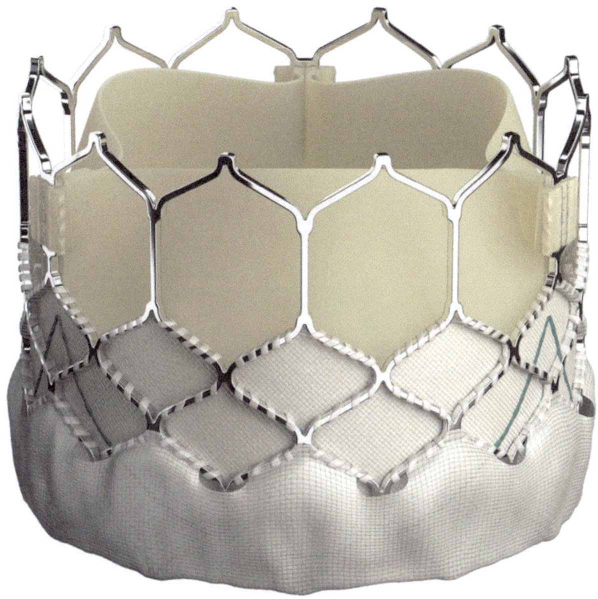

Fig. 8.1 Edwards Sapien 3 transcatheter aortic valve (Figure used with permission from Edwards Lifesciences Corporation, Irvine, CA, USA)

morbid patients presenting with hemodynamic instability where the contribution of the aortic stenosis to the overall condition is not clear.

BAV is usually performed as retrograde procedure via an arterial 10 or 12 French femoral access in conscious sedation. Rapid pacing during balloon inflation is recommendable. The choice of the balloon size (usually 20–23 mm) depends on the diameter of the aortic annulus, oversizing should be avoided.

Transcatheter valve replacement has been an experimental concept since 1965 [25]. From then it took another 25 years of stent technology development until the first percutaneous valve was implanted in a right ventricle to pulmonary artery prosthetic conduit in a young patient [26]. The first transcatheter aortic valve replacement followed in 2002 in an elderly male [27]. Since then transcatheter aortic valve replacement (TAVR) has shown a highly dynamic evolution. The initial devices have been re-designed several times and a considerable number of new devices are available now for commercial use in Europe (Fig. 8.1). At present there are basically three different technological principles used in biological transcatheter valves: valves are either mounted in balloon-expandable or self-expandable stents or in a polymeric tubing system which is expanded by fluid filling that is finally replaced by polymer.

The initial ante-grade access is still available as trans-apical procedure, the transseptal access however has been completely abandoned. At present the retrograde trans-femoral access is clearly predominant (Fig. 8.2). Occasional patients with a difficult femoral access are also done via a subclavian, direct aortic or carotid retrograde approach.

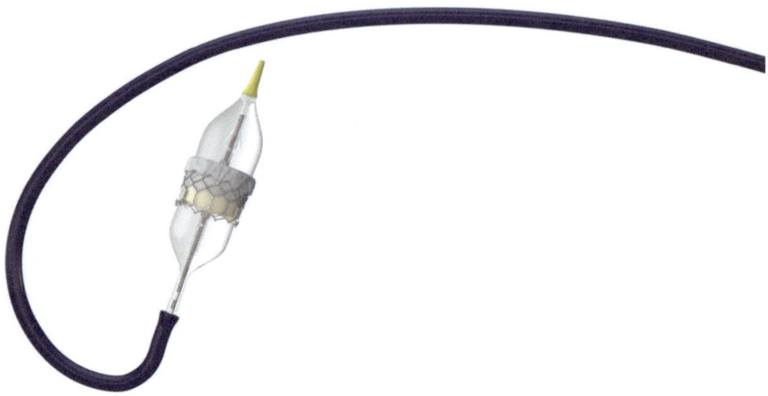

Fig. 8.2 Transfemoral delivery system "commander" for the Edwards Sapien 3 transcatheter valve (Figure used with permission from Edwards Lifesciences Corporation, Irvine, CA, USA)

Initial use of TAVR was restricted to elderly patients with high and very high surgical risk assessed by surgical risk scores as the Euroscore or the STS score [4, 5, 28]. It became clear that especially the Euroscore overestimated the surgical risk that is better predicted by the STS score [5, 29] and the Euroscore II [30]. However, STS and Euroscore II also neglect important risk determinants like frailty [31] Individual patient assessment by heart teams is therefore essential for patient selection.

Meanwhile two randomized landmark trials have confirmed the efficacy of TAVR with first generation transcatheter valves in patients with prohibitive surgical risk compared to medical therapy and in high risk patients compared to surgical valve replacement (SAVR). In the cohort B of the PARTNER trial 358 patients with aortic stenosis who were not considered to be suitable candidates for surgery underwent randomization to TAVR with the Edwards Sapien valve or standard therapy. Mean age of the cohort was 83 years and logistic Euroscore >20 %. One year mortality in the TAVR group was 30.7 % compared to 50.7 % in the group with standard therapy ($p<0.001$) [11]. In the cohort A of the PARTNER trial 699 high-risk patients (logistic Euroscore >20 %) with a mean age of 84 years were randomized to TAVR or SAVR. One year mortality in both groups was comparable (24.2 % for TAVR and 26.8 % for SAVR). The rate of stroke and vascular complications was higher with TAVR whereas major bleedings and atrial fibrillation occurred more often after SAVR [32]. The second first generation transcatheter valve, the CoreValve, was implanted in the U.S. CoreValve trial. The extreme risk group was a single arm registry of 506 patients with aortic-stenosis and prohibitive risks for surgery which showed a promising 24.3 % mortality and 4.3 % stroke rate after 1 year [33]. The high risk group consisted of 795 patients with a mean age of 83 years and a logistic Euroscore of approximately 18 %. Patients were randomized to TAVR with the Corevalve or SAVR. Mortality after 1 year was significantly lower in the TAVR compared to the SAVR cohort (14.2 % vs 19.1 %; p=0.04 for superiority) with no increased stroke rate (8.8 % versus 12.6 %) [34].

The better results of TAVR in the U.S. CoreValve trial compared to the PARTNER trial might be multi-factorial. Randomized data comparing different valve types are limited [35]. In spite of the fact that specific endpoints for TAVR trials have been defined (VARC and VARC II criteria) the short re-design cycles of these devices quickly invalidates such comparisons at present.

Paravalvular leaks, non-retrievability and access size have been felt to be the main shortcomings of the first generation devices. Paravalvular leaks have been associated with worse outcomes [36]. New device designs seem to be able to effectively reduce paravalvular leaks [37, 38]. Also other shortcomings are addressed [35].

Randomized comparisons of different access routes are lacking. Therefore any comparison of trans-apical and trans-femoral access is based on biased registry data with equivocal results. Patients' preference however seems to go for least invasive procedures with percutaneous closure of access site in conscious sedation. A transfer of TAVR therapy into lower risk populations is discussed very controversially.

The need for antiplatelets after the procedure for patients not on anticoagulation is not well defined. Many centres tend for long-term aspirin treatment and sometimes addition of clopidogrel for various time periods.

Transcatheter Valve Repair for Mitral Insufficiency

The most extensive experience on transcatheter therapy of mitral insufficiency exists for the MitraClip device (Abbott; Menlo Park, California) which is used for direct valve repair. In addition many other interventional approaches have been introduced including different annuloplasty procedures and transcatheter mitral valve replacement. The future relevance of these latter approaches is not yet clear. Therefore they are beyond the scope of this description.

Mitral insufficiency can originate from a primary abnormality of the valve, degenerative mitral regurgitation (DMR), or a functional abnormality secondary to left ventricular dysfunction, functional mitral regurgitation (FMR). In functional mitral regurgitation the underlying disease might be ischemic or non-ischemic. Obviously a long-standing DMR can cause left ventricular dysfunction leading to secondary FMR which results in a mixed situation.

Current American guidelines recommend surgery (especially mitral valve repair) for symptomatic patients with chronic severe mitral insufficiency due to a primary valvular abnormality as a class I indication whereas surgery for symptomatic patients with severe functional mitral insufficiency should only be considered as a class IIb indication [13]. The latter recommendation is based on the fact that the reported outcomes in this cohort of patients were equivocal.

The MitraClip system was developed on the basis of Alfieri's surgical edge-to-edge repair [39]. The clip (Fig. 8.3) is delivered percutaneously from the femoral

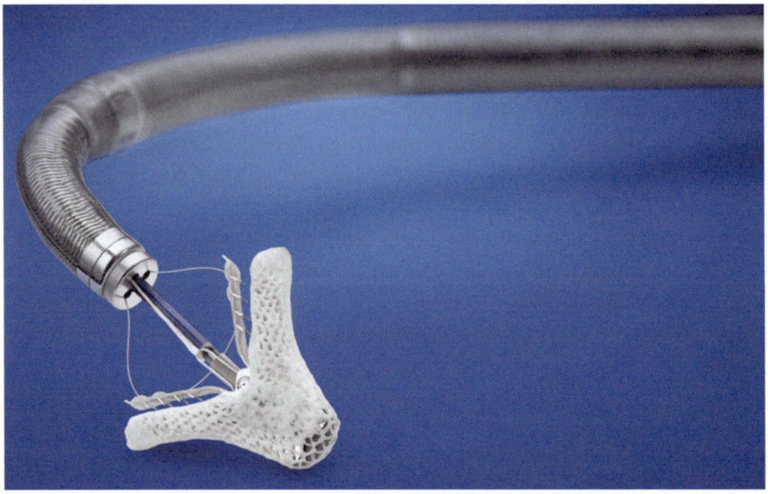

Fig. 8.3 MitraClip system for reduction of mitralregurgitation by approximating the anterior and posterior leaflets (Figure used with permission from Abbott Vascular, Santa Clara, CA, USA)

vein via a transseptal sheath under fluoroscopic and transoesophageal echocardiographic guidance. It reduces mitral regurgitation by approximating the anterior and posterior leaflets thus creating a double mitral valve orifice (Fig. 8.4). If necessary two or even more clips can be delivered in one session.

After safety and feasibility of the MitraClip system had been shown in the first in men single arm EVEREST I trial [40] it was compared in the multicentre, randomized EVEREST II trial against surgery (either replacement or repair) in patients with symptomatic severe mitral regurgitation who were also candidates for mitral valve surgery [41]. FMR was only present in 27 % of patients. Patients with severe LV dysfunction were excluded. Mitral regurgitation and NYHA class were significantly reduced in both groups. However, in the as treated analysis surgery more effectively reduced mitral regurgitation than the MitraClip (4 % vs 19 % residual high degree mitral insufficiency). Major adverse cardiac events after 30 days were comparable between groups. After 4 years 25 % of patients in the percutaneous repair group vs 5.5 % in the surgical group had undergone redo surgery for significant mitral regurgitation [42].

Thus the MitraClip is no alternative to surgery in patients who are low-risk candidates for surgery but in those who are deemed to be at high surgical risk. This was confirmed in several registries and applied to degenerative as well as functional etiologies [43, 44].

Recently a pooled analysis of 16 studies with a total of 2980 patients of whom 2689 were considered high-risk for surgery showed a low incidence of procedural death (0.1 %). Thirty day mortality was 4.2 % which compares very favourably to historical surgical data.

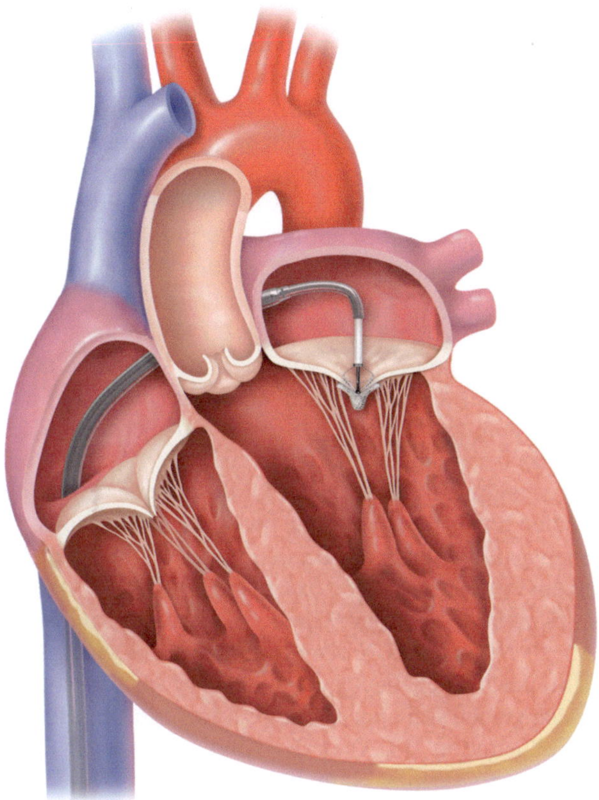

Fig. 8.4 Mode of implantation of the MitracClip system via transfemoral access (Figure used with permission from Abbott Vascular, Santa Clara, CA, USA)

Atrial Septal Defect Closure

Patients with significant atrial septal defects (ASD) frequently remain asymptomatic until adulthood. A majority only develops symptoms beyond the fourth decade. Therefore freedom from symptoms (e.g. reduced functional capacity, exertional shortness of breath, palpitations due to supraventricular arrhythmias, right heart failure) is no reliable predictor of a further benign course even in an elderly patient. A significant left to right shunt is usually defined as a pulmonary to systemic flow ratio (Q_P: Q_S) > 1.5. This ratio is however not only dependent on defect size but also on the LA to RA pressure gradient which is influenced by right and left ventricular compliance as well as pulmonary resistance. Left to right shunt can increase with decreasing left ventricular compliance (e.g. due to co-morbidities like arterial hypertension) or decrease with increasing pulmonary resistance. So a Q_P: Q_S < 1.5 does not exclude a significant ASD with preceding higher shunt volume. Therefore the 2010 ESC guideline on the management of grown-up congenital heart disease recommend to define a significant shunt rather based on signs of right ventricular volume overload [45]. A defect diameter of less than 10 mm with signs of right heart failure should however always raise suspicion on a causal relationship. In these cases an abnormal pulmonary venous connection has to be excluded.

It has been shown that surgical closure of significant ASD's beyond the age of 40 years might have a small mortality but definitely a good symptomatic effect compared to medical treatment [46]. Mortality after transcatheter closure is comparable to surgical closure. Morbidity is however higher with the surgical approach [47, 48]. This might be even more pronounced in the elderly.

Defect closure does not lower the frequency of arrhythmia during follow up in the elderly patient [46, 49]. If ablation of atrial fibrillation or flutter is considered this might therefore be performed before defect closure. Peri-interventional atrial fibrillation is however frequently self-limiting.

European guidelines recommend closure of all atrial septal defects with significant shunt as defined by right ventricular volume overload regardless of symptoms and as long as pulmonary vascular resistence is still less than 5 Wood units. ASD occlusion should also be considered if paradoxical embolism is suspected. No special recommendation is given for the elderly. Transcatheter closure is the preferred method if technically feasible. In patients with modestly increased pulmonary resistance an individualized decision has to be taken considering the response on vasodilators (preferably nitric oxide) [45].

A number of different devices suitable for transcatheter closure of atrial septal defects has gained CE mark over the recent years. A detailed technical description of all the different devices would be beyond the scope of this book. The only device which gained full approval for clinical use from the United States Food and Drug Administration (FDA) is the Amplatzer Septal Occluder (ASO). It is also the device with the most complete study results. The ASO is a self-expandable double-disk device made of nitinol which is connected by a 3–4 mm waist between the two disks with the left disk being larger than the right. A total of three Dacron polyester patches is sewn into each disk and the connecting waist. The device size is determined by the diameter of its waste and currently available from 4 to 38 mm. The device is released from a venous sheath which is advanced from the right atrium via the defect into the left atrium. After release of the left atrial disk the waste is released in the defect which self-centres the device before release of the right atrial disk (Fig. 8.5).

Transcatheter closure can only be considered in secundum ASD, which makes up for about 80 % of all ASD's. With primum ASD (15 %), superior sinus venosus defect (5 %), inferior sinus venosus defect (<1 %) and unroofed coronary sinus as well as in patients with abnormal pulmonary venous connections a surgical closure has to be performed. Before transcatheter closure of secundum ASD a transoesophageal echo is mandatory to look for the pulmonary venous connection and the tissue rim around the atrial septal defect. The rim should be at least 5 mm of adequate quality except towards the aorta. In addition the defect should not be bigger than 36–38 mm [45]. Interventional closure of large ASD's requires special technical skills and equipment (e.g. Hausdorf sheath).

When closing ASD's in elderly patients with more co-morbidities special consideration should be given to impaired systolic or diastolic function. The acute volume

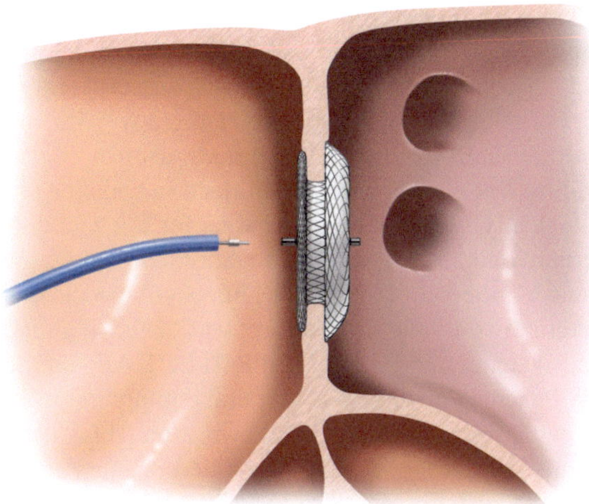

Fig. 8.5 Release of the Amplatzer Septal Occluder (Figure used with permission from St. Jude Medical GmbH, St Paul, MN, USA)

challenge of the left ventricle after the closure might increase the end-diastolic pressure to an extent that pulmonary oedema results. Precautions should be taken when the atrial filling pressure before closure is above 15 mmHg. A test occlusion of the ASD with the sizing balloon can be performed monitoring the atrial pressures via the wire lumen over 10–15 min. If the left atrial pressure increases by more than 5 mmHg closure should be postponed and patients pretreated with diuretics and after-load reduction before a further closure attempt with initial repetition of the left atrial pressure measurements. In some cases a fenestrated occluder might be considered [50].

In elderly in whom no interventional closure can be performed an individual risk benefit analysis should be performed before surgical closure taking into account the individual co-morbidities [45].

After the procedure a minimum of 6 month aspirin treatment at a dose of 100 mg is recommended. Many centres add 75 mg clopidogrel for a variable time. Endocarditis prophylaxis is recommended during the first 6 month after device implantation [45].

Left Atrial Appendage Closure

The concept of left atrial appendage (LAA) closure for stroke prevention in atrial fibrillation is based on the observation that more than 90 % of emboli seem to originate from the left atrial appendage [51]. Surgical closure with different techniques have been done for several years; nevertheless the mainly non-randomized data were equivocal [52, 53].

Technical feasibility of interventional occlusion via a transseptal sheath was first shown in 2001 with the dedicated Plaato device which is no longer commercially available [54]. Shortly afterwards occlusion procedures with non-dedicated Amplatzer devices were reported [55]. These first procedures were predominantly done in patients with contra-indications to oral anticoagulation. After the procedure patients received dual antiplatelet therapy with aspirin and clopidogrel for 1–6 months usually followed by lifelong aspirin. With respect to the non-negligible bleeding risk also aspirin was stopped in some patients after 6 months.

Basically two different scenarios for LAA occlusion have to be considered: as alternative to anticoagulation when oral anticoagulation is possible and as replacement for anticoagulation when anticoagulation is not possible.

Actually only the first concept was tested in a randomized fashion with the dedicated Watchman device in the PROTECT AF and the PREVAIL studies. In spite of early hazards due to peri-procedural complications equivalence to oral anticoagulation with warfarin could be shown after 1065 patient years of follow-up in 707 patients with respect to the combined primary endpoint of stroke, cardiovascular death and systemic enbolisation (3.0 vs 4.9 events per 100 patient years) and superiority after 2621 patient years of follow-up (2.3 vs 3.8 events per 100 patient years) in the PROTECT AF trial [56, 57]. The interventional LAA occlusion in the PROTECT AF trial was followed by warfarin treatment for another 45 days which should be replaced by clopidogrel up to 6 month if transoesophageal echo did not show thrombus formation on the device. Warfarin and clopidogrel were given in combination with aspirin that was recommended for lifelong therapy. After 45 days and 2 years a vast majority of patients in the device group (87 % rsp. 94 %) had actually abandoned warfarin therapy. The PROTECT AF results were confirmed by the PREVAIL trial which also showed a significant reduction of peri-procedural complications (e.g. perforation, stroke, device embolization) compared to the PROTECT AF trial probably due to increasing operator experience [58]. Non-surprisingly the average age of the studied population in both trials was above 70 years what reflects the increasing prevalence of atrial fibrillation and embolic stroke risk with age.

A current consensus statement from the European Society of Cardiology is still reluctant to generally recommend LAA occlusion as alternative to anticoagulation when anticoagulation is possible [59]. The main arguments are that the early interventional hazards with device closure are significant especially at the beginning of the learning curve which is deemed to be rather slow compared to other interventions. Furthermore the main advantage of LAA closure compared to vitamin K antagonists seems to be the reduction of hemorrhagic strokes which might also be achieved with the novel oral anticoagulants that have not been compared yet to LAA device occlusion. Nevertheless the Watchman device recently gained approval for this indication from the United States Food and Drug Administration (FDA).

The focus of the current European consensus statement is rather on replacement of anticoagulation when anticoagulation is not possible. It has to be clearly stated that this indication is only based on registry data and non-randomized comparisons to historical stroke-rates or calculated stroke-rates according to established risk scores. Of the four CE marked devices the Watchman, the ACP including the newest

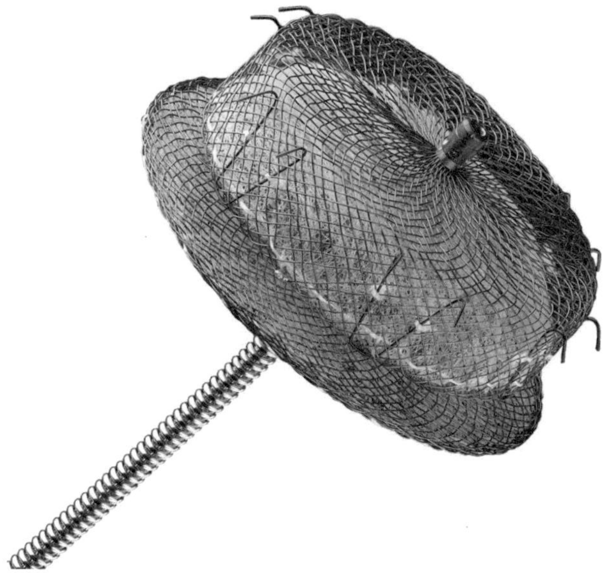

Fig. 8.6 Amplatzer Cardiac Plug (Figure used with permission from St. Jude Medical GmbH, St Paul, MN, USA)

Amulet generation and the Wavecrest aim at a mechanical device obstruction of the LAA via a purely endocardial approach whereas the Lariat device is used for a endocardial/epicardial suture ligation. Most data are available for the Watchman and the ACP (Fig. 8.6). For both devices registries have been performed without post-interventional anticoagulation but dual antiplatelet therapy for 1–6 months followed by indefinite aspirin therapy [60, 61]. Cessation of aspirin after 6 months was also reported [59].

References

1. Jung B, Baron G, Butchart EG, Delahaye F, Gohlke-Bärwolf C, Levang OW, Tornos P, Vanoverschelde JL, Vermeer F, Boersma E, Ravaud P, Vahanian A. A prospective survey of patients with valvular heart disease in Europe: the Euro Heart Survey on valvular heart disease. Eur Heart J. 2003;24:1231–43.
2. Jang SY, Ju EY, Seo SR, Choi JY, Park SJ, Kim DK, Park SW. Changes in the etiology of valvular heart disease in the rapidly aging Korean population. Int J Cardiol. 2014;174:355–9.
3. Carabello RA, Paulus WJ. Aortic stenosis. Lancet. 2009;373:956–66.
4. Nashef SA, Roques F, Sharples LD, Nilsson J, Smith C, Goldstone AR, Lockowandt U. EuroSCORE II. Eur J Cardiothorac Surg. 2012;41:734–44.
5. Wendt D, Osswald BR, Kayser K, Thielmann M, Tossios P, Massoudy P, Karnler M, Jacob H. Society of Thoracic Surgeons score is superior to the EuroSCORE determining mortality in high risk patients undergoing isolated aortic valve replacement. Ann Thorac Surg. 2009;88: 468–78.
6. Mirabel M, Jung B, Baron G, Messika-Zeitoun D, Détain D, Vanoverschelde JL, Butchart EG, Ravaud P, Vahanian A. What are the characteristics of patients with severe, symptomatic, mitral regurgitation who are denied surgery? Eur Heart J. 2007;28:1358–65.

7. Long T, Lopez BM, Berberian C, Cunningham MJ, Starnes VA, Cohen RG. Exercise hemodynamics and quality of life after aortic valve replacement for aortic stenosis in the elderly using the Hancock II bioprosthesis. Cardiol Res Pract. 2014;2014:151282. doi:10.1155/2014/151282. Epub 2014 Dec 2.
8. Bekelman DB, Rumsfeld JS, Havranek EP, Yamashita TE, Hutt E, Gottlieb SH, Kutner JS. Symptom burden, depression, and spiritual well-being: a comparison of heart failure and advanced cancer patients. J Gen Intern Med. 2009;24:592–8.
9. Lieberman EB, Bashore TM, Hermiller JB, Wilson JS, Pieper KS, Keeler GP, Pierce CH, Kisslo KB, Harrison JK, Davidson CJ. Balloon aortic valvuloplasty in adults: failure of procedure to improve long-term survival. J Am Coll Cardiol. 1995;26:1522–8.
10. Safian RD, Berman AD, Diver DJ, McKay LL, Come PC, Riley MF, Warren SE, Cunningham MJ, Wyman RM, Weinstein JS. Balloon aortic valvuloplasty in 170 consecutive patients. N Engl J Med. 1988;19:125–30.
11. Leon MB, Smith CR, Mack M, Miller DC, Moses JW, Svensson LG, Tuzcu EM, Webb JG, Fontana GP, Makkar RR, Brown DL, Block PC, Guyton RA, Pichard AD, Bavaria JE, Herrmann HC, Douglas PS, Petersen JL, Akin JJ, Anderson WN, Wang D, Pocock S, PARTNER Trial Investigators. Transcatheter aortic-valve implantation for aortic stenosis in patients who cannot undergo surgery. N Engl J Med. 2010;363:1597–607.
12. Beigel R, Wunderlich NC, Kar S, Siegel RJ. The evolution of percutaneous mitral valve repair therapy: lessons learned and implications for patient selection. J Am Coll Cardiol. 2014;64:2688–700.
13. Nishimura RA, Otto CM, Bonow RO, Carabello BA, 3rd Erwin JP, Guyton RA, O'Gara PT, Ruiz CE, Skubas NJ, Sorajja P, 3rd Sundt TM, Thomas JD, Anderson JL, Halperin JL, Albert NM, Bozkurt B, Brindis RG, Creager MA, Curtis LH, DeMets D, Guyton RA, Hochman JS, Kovacs RJ, Ohman EM, Pressler SJ, Sellke FW, Shen WK, Stevenson WG, Yancy CW, American College of Cardiology; American College of Cardiology/American Heart Association; American Heart Association. 2014 AHA/ACC guideline for the management of patients with valvular heart disease: a report of the American College of Cardiology/American Heart Association Task Force on Practice Guidelines. J Thorac Cardiovasc Surg. 2014; 148:e1–132.
14. Block PC, Burstein S, Casale PN, Kramer PH, Teirstein P, Williams DO, Reisman M. Percutaneous left atrial appendage occlusion for patients in atrial fibrillation suboptimal for warfarin therapy: 5-year results of the PLAATO (Percutaneous Left Atrial Appendage Transcatheter Occlusion) Study. JACC Cardiovasc Interv. 2009;2:594–600.
15. Reddy VY, Holmes D, Doshi SK, Neuzil P, Kar S. Safety of percutaneous left atrial appendage closure: results from the Watchman Left Atrial Appendage System for Embolic Protection in Patients with AF (PROTECT AF) clinical trial and the Continued Access Registry. Circulation. 2011;123:417–24.
16. Genders TS, Steyerberg EW, Hunink MG, Nieman K, Galema TW, Mollet NR, de Feyter PJ, Krestin GP, Alkadhi H, Leschka S, Desbiolles L, Meijs MF, Cramer MJ, Knuuti J, Kajander S, Bogaert J, Goetschalckx K, Cademartiri F, Maffei E, Martini C, Seitun S, Aldrovandi A, Wildermuth S, Stinn B, Fornaro J, Feuchtner G, De Zordo T, Auer T, Plank F, Friedrich G, Pugliese F, Petersen SE, Davies LC, Schoepf UJ, Rowe GW, van Mieghem CA, van Driessche L, Sinitsyn V, Gopalan D, Nikolaou K, Bamberg F, Cury RC, Battle J, Maurovich-Horvat P, Bartykowszki A, Merkely B, Becker D, Hadamitzky M, Hausleiter J, Dewey M, Zimmermann E, Laule M. Prediction model to estimate presence of coronary artery disease: retrospective pooled analysis of existing cohorts. BMJ. 2012;344, e3485.
17. Brunner KJ, Bunch TJ, Mullin CM, May HAT, Bair TL, Elliot DW, Anderson JL, Mahapatra S. Clinical predictors of risk for atrial fibrillation: implications for diagnosis and monitoring. Mayo Clin Proc. 2014;89:1498–505.
18. Lip GY, Frison L, Halperin JL, Dane DA. Comparative validation of a novel risk score for predicting bleeding risk in anticoagulated patients with atrial fibrillation: the HAS-BLED (Hypertension, Abnormal Renal/Liver Function, Stroke, Bleeding History or Predisposition, Labile INR, Elderly, Drugs/Alcohol Concomitantly) score. J Am Coll Cardiol. 2011;57:173–80.

19. Varadarajan P, Kapoor N, Bansal RC, Pai RG. Clinical profile and natural history of 453 non-surgically managed patients with severe aortic stenosis. Ann Thorac Surg. 2006;82:2111–5.
20. Bach DS, Siao D, Girard SE, Duvernoy C, McCallister Jr BD, Gualano SK. Evaluation of patients with severe symptomatic aortic stenosis who do not undergo aortic valve replacement: the potential role of subjectively overestimated operative risk. Circ Cardiovasc Qual Outcomes. 2009;2:533–9.
21. Ross Jr J, Braunwald E. The influence of corrective operations on the natural history of aortic stenosis. Circulation. 1968;38(1 Suppl):61–7.
22. Frank S, Johnson A, Ross Jr J. Natural history of valvular aortic stenosis. Br Heart J. 1973;35:41–6.
23. Cribier A, Savin T, Saoudi N, Rocha P, Berland J, Lelac B. Percutaneous transluminal valvuloplasty of acquired aortic stenosis in elderly patients: an alternative to valve replacement? Lancet. 1986;1:63–7.
24. National Heart Lung and Blood Institute participants group. Percutaneous balloon aortic valvuloplasty. Acute and 30-day follow-up results in 674 patients from the NHLBI Balloon Valvuloplasty Registry. Circulation. 1991;84:2383–97.
25. Davies H. Catheter mounted valve for temporary relief of aortic insufficiency. Lancet. 1965;1:926–9.
26. Bonhoeffer P, Boudjemline Y, Saliba Z, Merckx J, Aggoun Y, Bonnet D, Acar P, Le Bidois J, Sidi D, Kachaner J. Percutaneous replacement of pulmonary valve in a right-ventricle to pulmonary-artery prosthetic conduit with valve dysfunction. Lancet. 2000;356:1403–5.
27. Cribier A, Eltchaninoff H, Bash A, Borenstein N, Tron C, Bauer F, Derumeaux G, Anselme F, Laborde F, Leon MB. Percutaneous transcatheter implantation of an aortic valve prosthesis for calcific aortic stenosis: first human case description. Circulation. 2002;10:3006–8.
28. Cribier A, Eltchaninoff H, Tron C, Bauer F, Agatiello C, Sebagh L, Bash A, Nusimovici D, Litzler PY, Bessou JP, Leon MB. Early experience with percutaneous transcatheter implantation of heart valve prosthesis for the treatment of end-stage inoperable patients with calcific aortic stenosis. J Am Coll Cardiol. 2004;43:698–703.
29. Hamm CW, Möllmann H, Holzhey D, Beckmann A, Veit C, Figulla HR, Cremer J, Kuck KH, Lange R, Zahn R, Sack S, Schuler G, Walther T, Beyersdorf F, Böhm M, Heusch G, Funkat AK, Neumann T, Papoutsis K, Schneider S, Welz A, Mohr FW, GARY-Executive Board. The German Aortic Valve Registry (GARY): in-hospital outcome. Eur Heart J. 2014;35:1588–98.
30. Holinski S, Jessen S, Neumann K, Konnertz W. Predictive Power and Implication of EuroSCORE, EuroSCORE II and STS Score for Isolated Repeated Aortic Valve Replacement. Ann Thorac Cardiovasc Surg. 2015;21:242–6.
31. Green P, Woglom AE, Genereux P, Daneault P, Paradis JM, Schnell S, Hawkey M, Maurer MS, Kirtane AJ, Kodali S, Moses JW, Leon MB, Smith CR, Williams M. The impact of frailty status on survival after transcatheter aortic valve replacement in older adults with severe aortic stenosis: a single-center experience. JACC Cardiovasc Interv. 2012;5:974–81.
32. Smith CR, Leon MB, Mack MJ, Miller DC, Moses JW, Svensson LG, Tuzcu EM, Webb JG, Fontana GP, Makkar RR, Williams M, Dewey T, Kapadia S, Babaliaros V, Thourani VH, Corso P, Pichard AD, Bavaria JE, Herrmann HC, Akin JJ, Anderson WN, Wang D, Pocock SJ, PARTNER Trial Investigators. Transcatheter versus surgical aortic-valve replacement in high-risk patients. N Engl J Med. 2011;364:2187–98.
33. Popma JJ, Adams DH, Reardon MJ, Yakubov SJ, Kleiman NS, Heimansohn D, Hermiller Jr J, Hughes GC, Harrison JK, Corselli J, Diez J, Kafi A, Schreiber T, Gleason TG, Conte J, Buchbinder M, Deeb GM, Carabello B, Serruys PW, Chenoweth S, Oh JK, CoreValve United States Investigators. Transcatheter aortic valve replacement using a self-expanding bioprosthesis in patients with severe aortic stenosis at extreme risk for surgery. J Am Coll Cardiol. 2014;63:1972–81.
34. Adams DH, Popma JJ, Reardon MJ, Yakubov SJ, Coselli JS, Deeb GM, Gleason TG, Buchbinder M, Hermiller Jr J, Kleiman NS, Chetcuti S, Heiser J, Merhi W, Zorn G, Tadros P, Robinson M, Petrossian G, Hughes GC, Harrison JK, Conte J, Maini B, Mumtaz M, Chenoweth S, Oh JK, U.S. CoreValve Clinical Investigators. Transcatheter aortic-valve replacement with a self-expanding prosthesis. N Engl J Med. 2014;370:1790–8.

35. Abdel-Wahab M, Mehilli J, Frerker C, Neumann FJ, Kurz T, Tölg R, Zachow D, Guerra E, Massberg S, Schäfer U, El-Mawardy M, Richardt G, CHOICE investigators. Comparison of balloon-expandable vs self-expandable valves in patients undergoing transcatheter aortic valve replacement: the CHOICE randomized clinical trial. JAMA. 2014;311:1503–14.
36. Genereux P, Head SJ, Hahn R, Daneault B, Kodali S, Williams MR, van Mieghem NM, Alu MC, Serruys PW, Kappetein AP, Leon MB. Paravalvular leak after transcatheter aortic valve replacement: the new Achilles' heel? A comprehensive review of the literature. J Am Coll Cardiol. 2013;61:1125–36.
37. Meredith IT, Walters DL, Dumonteil N, Worthley SG, Tchetche D, Manoharan G, Blackman DJ, Rioufol G, Hildick-Smith D, Whitbourn RJ, Lefevre T, Lange R, Müller R, Redwood S, Alloco DJ, Dawkins KD. Transcatheter aortic valve replacement for severe symptomatic aortic stenosis using a repositionable valve system: 30-day primary endpoint results from the REPRISE II study. J Am Coll Cardiol. 2014;64:1339–48.
38. Webb J, Gerosa G, Lefevre T, Leipsic J, Spence M, Thomas M, Thielmann M, Treede H, Wendler O, Walther T. Multicenter evaluation of a next-generation balloon-expandable transcatheter aortic valve. J Am Coll Cardiol. 2014;64:2235–43.
39. Maisano F, Schreuder JJ, Oppizzi M, Florani B, Fino C, Alfieri O. The double-orifice technique as a standardized approach to treat mitral regurgitation due to sever myxomatous disease: surgical technique. Eur J Cardiothorac Surg. 2000;17:201–5.
40. Feldman T, Kar S, Rinaldi M, Fail P, Hermiller J, Smalling R, Whitlow PL, Gray W, Low R, Herrman HC, Lim S, Foster E, Glower D, EVEREST Investigators. Percutaneous mitral repair with the MitraClip system: safety and midtern durability in the initial EVEREST (Endovascular Valve Edge-to-Edge Repair Study) cohort. J Am Coll Cardiol. 2009;54:686–94.
41. Feldman T, Foster E, Glower DD, Kar S, Rinaldi MJ, Fail PS, Smalling RW, Siegel R, Rose GA, Engeron G, Loghin C, Trento A, Skipper ER, Fudge T, Letsou GV, Massaro JM, Mauri L, EVEREST II Investigators. Percutaneous repair or surgery for mitral regurgitation. N Engl J Med. 2011;364:1395–406.
42. Mauri L, Foster E, Glower DD, Apruzzesse P, Massaro JM, Herrmann HC, Hermiller J, Gray W, Wang A, Pedersen WR, Bajwa T, Lasala J, Low R, Grayburn P, Feldman T, Everest II Investigators. 4-year results of a randomized controlled trial of percutaneous repair versus surgery for mitral regurgitation. J Am Coll Cardiol. 2013;62:317–28.
43. Whitlow PL, Feldman T, Pedersen WR, Lim DS, Kipperman R, Smalling R, Bajwa T, Herrmann HC, Lasala J, Maddux JT, Tuczu M, Kapadia S, Trento A, Siegel RJ, Foster E, Glower D, Mauri L, Kar S, Everest II Investigators. Acute and 12-month results with catheter-based mitral valve leaflet repair: the EVEREST II (Endovascular Valve Edge-to-Edge Repair) High Risk Study. J Am Coll Cardiol. 2012;59:130–9.
44. Maisano F, Franzen O, Baldus S, Schäfer U, Hausleiter J, Butter C, Ussia GP, Sievert H, Richardt G, Widder JD, Moccetti T, Schillinger W. Percutaneous mitral valve interventions in the real world: early and 1-year results from the ACCESS EU, a prospective, multicenter, nonrandomized post-approval study of the MitraClip therapy in Europe. J Am Coll Cardiol. 2013;17:1052–61.
45. Baumgärtner H, Bonhoeffer P, de Groot NMS, de Haan F, Deanfield JE, Galie N, Gatzoulis MA, Gohlke-Baerwolf C, Kaemmerer H, Kilner P, Meijboom F, Mulder BJM, Oechslin E, Oliver JM, Serraf A, Szatmari A, Thaulow E, Vouhe PR, Walma E. ESC Guidelines for the management of grown-up congenital heart disease. Eur Heart J. 2010;31:2915–57.
46. Attie F, Rosas M, Granados N, Zabal C, Buendia A, Calderon J. Surgical treatment for secundum atrial septal defects in patients>40 years old. J Am Coll Cardiol. 2001;38:2035–42.
47. Du ZD, Hijazi ZM, Kleinmann CS, Silvermann NH, Larntz K. Comparison between transcatheter and surgical closure of secundum atrial septal defect in children and adults: results of a multicenter nonrandomized trial. J Am Coll Cardiol. 2002;39:1836–44.
48. Butera G, Carminati M, Chessa M, Youssef R, Drago M, Giamberti A, Pome G, Bossone E, Frigola A. Percutaneous versus surgical closure of secundum atrial septal defect: comparison of early results and complications. Am Heart J. 2006;151:228–34.

49. Humenberger M, Rosenhek R, Gabriel H, Radar F, Heger M, Klaar U, Binder T, Probst P, Heinze G, Maurer G, Baumgartner H. Benefit of atrial septal defect closure in adults: impact of age. Eur Heart J. 2010;32:553–60.
50. Al-Hindi A, Cao QL, Hijazi ZM. Transcatheter closure of atrial septal defect in the elderly. J Invasive Cardiol. 2009;21:70–5.
51. Blackshear J, Odell J. Appendage obliteration to reduce stroke in cardiac surgical patients with atrial fibrillation. Ann Thorac Surg. 1996;61:755–9.
52. Kanderian AS, Gillinov AM, Petterson GB, Blackstone E, Klein AL. Success of surgical left atrial appendage closure: assessment by transesophageal echocardiography. J Am Coll Cardiol. 2008;52:924–9.
53. Friedman PA, Asirvatham S, Dalegrave C, Kinoshita M, Danielsen AJ, Johnson SB, Hodge DO, Munger TM, Packer DL, Bruce CJ. Percutaneous epicardial left atrial appendage closure: preliminary results of an electrogram guided approach. J Cardiovasc Electrophysiol. 2009;20: 908–15.
54. Sievert H, Lesh M, Trepels T, Omran H, Bartorelli A, Della Bella P, Nakai T, Reisman M, DiMario C, Block P, Kramer P, Fleschenberg D, Krumsdorf U, Scherer D. Percutaneous left atrial appendage transcatheter occlusion to prevent stroke in high-risk patients with atrial fibrillation: early clinical experience. Circulation. 2002;105:1887–9.
55. Meier B, Palacios I, Windecker S, Rotter M, Cao QL, Keane D, Ruiz CE, Hijazi ZM. Transcatheter left atrial appendage occlusion with Amplatzer devices to obviate anticoagulation in patients with atrial fibrillation. Catheter Cardiovasc Interv. 2003;60:417–22.
56. Holmes DR, Reddy VY, Turi ZG, Doshi SK, Sievert H, Buchbinder M, Mullin CM, Sick P, PROTECT AF Investigators. Percutaneous closure of the left atrial appendage versus warfarin therapy for prevention of stroke in patients with atrial fibrillation: a randomised non-inferiority trial. Lancet. 2009;374:534–42.
57. Reddy VY, Sievert H, Halperin J, Doshi SK, Buchbinder M, Neuzil P, Huber K, Whisenant B, Kar S, Swarup V, Gordon N, Holmes D, PROTECT AF Steering Committee and Investigators. Percutaneous left atrial appendage closure vs warfarin for atrial fibrillation: a randomized clinical trial. JAMA. 2014;312:1988–98.
58. Holmes Jr DR, Kar S, Price MJ, Whisenant B, Sievert H, Doshi SK, Huber K, Reddy VY. Prospective randomized evaluation of the Watchman left atrial appendage closure device in patients with atrial fibrillation versus long-term warfarin therapy: the PREVAIL trial. J Am Coll Cardiol. 2014;64:1–12.
59. Meier B, Blaauw Y, Khattab AA, Lewalter T, Sievert H, Tondo C, Glikson M, Document Reviewers. EHRA/EAPCI expert consensus statement on catheter-based left atrial appendage occlusion. Europace. 2014;16:1397–416.
60. Reddy VY, Möbius-Winkler S, Miller MA, Neuzil P, Schuler G, Wiebe J, Sick P, Sievert H. Left atrial appendage closure with the Watchman device in patients with a contraindication for oral anticoagulation: the ASAP study (ASA Plavix Feasibility Study With Watchman Left Atrial Appendage Closure Technology). J Am Coll Cardiol. 2013;61:2551–6.
61. Park JW, Bethencourt A, Sievert H, Santoro G, Meier B, Walsh K, Lopez-Minguez JR, Meerkin D, Valdes M, Omerod O, Leithäuser B. Left atrial appendage closure with Amplatzer cardiac plug in atrial fibrillation: Initial European experience. Catheter Cardiovasc Interv. 2011;77:700–6.

Chapter 9
Pulmonary Hypertension in the Elderly: Impact of Age on Diagnosis and Therapy Options

Tobias J. Lange

Definition of Pulmonary Hypertension

Pulmonary hypertension (PH) is defined by a mean pulmonary artery pressure (mPAP) $\geq$25 mmHg at rest on right heart catheterization (RHC) regardless of age [1]. This definition is based on historical consensus and a large number of RHC data in healthy subjects who show a mean mPAP of 14.0 mmHg with a standard deviation (SD) of about 3 mmHg at rest which is hardly influenced by body position and sex [2]. In older people ($\geq$50 years) the mean mPAP at rest was slightly higher compared to people aged 30–50 years (14.7 vs. 12.9 mmHg, $p<0.001$), which was regarded to be negligible with respect to hemodynamic PH definition [1, 2]. However, already on slight exercise the difference in mean mPAP between older and younger people became considerably wide (29.4 vs. 20.0 mmHg, $p<0.001$) with about 47 % of older people exceeding an mPAP of 30 mmHg [2]. Therefore the exercise definition of PH (mPAP > 30 mmHg) has been abandoned at the 4th World Symposium on PH in 2008 [3].

The pulmonary artery wedge pressure (PAWP) is used to define a precapillary (PAWP $\leq$ 15 mmHg) and a postcapillary form of PH (PAWP > 15 mmHg) at rest [1]. While in a large review of RHC data no relevant difference in PAWP between older and younger healthy subjects has been found at rest, older people showed a steeper increase in PAWP on exercise, which led to higher mPAP [2]. Another factor influencing PAWP (and mPAP) is the amount of intravascular fluid. On the one hand rapid saline infusions can lead to an increase in PAWP > 15 mmHg even in healthy subjects, on the other hand patients with left heart diseases (especially heart failure with preserved ejection fraction, HFpEF) can show PAWP of $\leq$15 mmHg at rest (e.g., after intensive diuretic treatment) [4]. Even if currently

T.J. Lange
Department of Internal Medicine II, University Medical Center Regensburg, Regensburg, Germany
e-mail: tobias.lange@ukr.de

H. Rittger (ed.), *Interventional Cardiology in the Elderly*,
DOI 10.1007/978-3-319-21142-8_9

there is no consensus on a definition of exercise-induced PH and no standardized fluid loading protocol to unmask latent left heart disease, these facts should be kept in mind when interpreting RHC measurements in patient populations at high risk for HFpEF (e.g. elderly patients).

Classification and Epidemiology of Pulmonary Hypertension

Since the 2nd Word Symposium on "primary PH" (PPH) in 1998, the PH classification system consists of five groups according to etiology, similar hemodynamic and clinical features, and therapeutic implications [5]. The current PH classification system [6], which has been slightly modified during the following PH World Symposia, is displayed in Table 9.1.

Group 1, Pulmonary Arterial Hypertension

The term "pulmonary arterial hypertension" (PAH) is restricted to describe group 1 of the classification system since 1998 [5]. Historically, PH of known causes ("secondary PH") was differentiated from PPH, which comprises the group of idiopathic, heritable, and anorexigen-associated PAH of the current classification system [7]. Today, PAH associated with connective tissue disease and other conditions is included (Table 9.1) [6]. PAH is characterized by a precapillary PH at rest on RHC (mPAP≥25 mmHg and PAWP≤15 mmHg) together with a pulmonary vascular resistance (PVR)>3 wood units (WU) [1]. Importantly, the diagnosis of PAH can only be made after accurate exclusion of known PH causes (groups 2–4) [8].

PAH is an orphan disease with an estimated incidence and prevalence of 2.0–7.6 and 10.6–26.0 cases per one million adult inhabitants, respectively [9]. The historically dismal prognosis with a median survival of less than 3 years from diagnosis has improved considerably over the recent years [10, 11]. With respect to age at diagnosis, we observed a considerable increase during the last 30 years. In the first US-based registry of PPH (sponsored by the National Institute of Health, therefore also called "NIH-registry") which recruited 187 patients between 1981 and 1985, the mean (± SD) age at diagnosis was 36 ± 15 years, while the mean age of 2525 patients enrolled in the current US registry of PAH (Registry to EValuate Early And Long-term pulmonary arterial hypertension disease management, REVEAL) was 53 ± 14 years [12, 13]. Of note, there are major differences in inclusion criteria between the NIH-registry and REVEAL as for example PAWP on RHC (≤12 vs. ≤ 15 mmHg) and the recruitment of prevalent patients in REVEAL. However, the trend of increasing age at diagnosis is also observed in other prospective registries (e.g., 50 ± 17 years in 482 incident patients with idiopathic, heritable, and anorexigen-associated PAH from United Kingdom and Ireland, recruited from 2001 to 2009) and clinical studies [14]. The so far reported

Table 9.1 Updated classification of pulmonary hypertension

1. Pulmonary arterial hypertension
1.1 Idiopathic PAH
1.2 Heritable PAH
1.2.1 BMPR2
1.2.2 ALK-1, ENG, SMAD9, CAV1, KCNK3
1.2.3 Unknown
1.3 Drug and toxin induced
1.4 Associated with:
1.4.1 Connective tissue disease
1.4.2 HIV infection
1.4.3 Portal hypertension
1.4.4 Congenital heart diseases
1.4.5 Schistosomiasis
1′ Pulmonary veno-occlusive disease and/or pulmonary capillary hemangiomatosis
1″ Persistent pulmonary hypertension of the newborn (PPHN)
2. Pulmonary hypertension due to left heart disease
2.1 Left ventricular systolic dysfunction
2.2 Left ventricular diastolic dysfunction
2.3 Valvular disease
2.4 Congenital/acquired left heart inflow/outflow tract obstruction and congenital cardiomyopathies
3. Pulmonary hypertension due to lung diseases and/or hypoxia
3.1 Chronic obstructive pulmonary disease
3.2 Interstitial lung disease
3.3 Other pulmonary diseases with mixed restrictive and obstructive pattern
3.4 Sleep-disordered breathing
3.5 Alveolar hypoventilation disorders
3.6 Chronic exposure to high altitude
3.7 Developmental lung diseases
4. Chronic thromboembolic pulmonary hypertension (CTEPH)
5. Pulmonary hypertension with unclear multifactorial mechanisms
5.1 Hematologic disorders: chronic hemolytic anemia, myeloproliferative disorders, splenectomy
5.2 Systemic disorders: sarcoidosis, pulmonary histiocytosis, lymphangioleiomyomatosis
5.3 Metabolic disorders: glycogenstorage disease, Gaucher disease, thyroiddisorders
5.4 Others: tumoral obstruction, fibrosing mediastinitis, chronic renal failure, segmental PH

From Ref. [6]

BMPR bone morphogenic protein receptor type II, *CAV1* caveolin-1, *ENG* endoglin, *HIV* human immunodeficiency virus, *PAH* pulmonary arterial hypertension

highest median age of 71 years in 587 patients with idiopathic PAH comes from a current analysis of the Comparative, Prospective Registry of Newly Initiated Therapies for Pulmonary Hypertension (COMPERA), which was launched in 2007 and is mainly fed by German PH centers [15].

Besides aging of the general populations of western countries, the main reason for this observation might be a change in referral pattern due to increased awareness of the disease in the face of steadily increasing medical treatment options. Interestingly, in countries with less or even no available PAH medications like China, the mean age at PAH diagnosis nowadays is about the age of patients at the time of the NIH registry [16]. However, the consequences of this demographic change in western countries are well described. Patients diagnosed with PAH at an older age have more comorbidities, less severe hemodynamics, worse functional status, and worse survival [13–15].

Major comorbidities in elderly patients (age > 50 years) with PAH which are significantly more common compared to younger patients are ischemic heart disease, arterial hypertension, atrial fibrillation, diabetes mellitus, and hypothyroidism [14]. In addition, even if not clearly related to age, obesity became more prevalent over time [13, 14]. The higher prevalence of mentioned comorbidities in elderly patients with PAH increases the complexity of differential diagnosis, and may lead to delayed PAH diagnosis in these patients [14]. On the other hand, elderly patients with HFpEF may be falsely diagnosed with PAH [1, 17, 18].

With respect to hemodynamic disease severity at diagnosis, elderly patients show a lower mean mPAP and a slightly but significantly higher mean PAWP at similar values for cardiac output, leading to a lower mean PVR [14, 15]. In an analysis from COMPERA, mPAP was even inversely correlated to age at diagnosis ($r = -0.44$, $p < 0.001$) [15]. These data could reflect a lower capacity of "older" right ventricles to compensate for increasing PVR. This could also explain that elderly patients are more symptomatic (as reflected by higher WHO functional class (FC)) and show a worse functional status (as reflected by lower exercise capacity) compared to younger patients [15]. In addition, clinical signs reflecting a worse right ventricular function like peripheral edema are more prevalent in elderly patients at PAH diagnosis [14]. Finally, elderly PAH patients show a worse survival compared to younger patients even after statistical correction for expected lower survival rates in older people from the general population [15].

Group 2, Pulmonary Hypertension Due to Left Heart Disease

Group 2 of the classification system covers PH due to left heart disease, which can be a consequence of heart failure with reduced as well as with preserved left ventricular function, aortic or mitral valve disease (see Table 9.1) [6]. Hemodynamically, PH in this group is usually postcapillary (PAWP > 15 mmHg) at rest, even if especially patients with HFpEF can show PAWP values ≤15 mmHg after intensive diuretic therapy [1, 18]. This should be considered when elderly patients with risk factors for HFpEF (e.g., obesity, arterial hypertension, atrial fibrillation etc.) are examined by RHC to avoid an overdiagnosis of PAH. Slight exercise or fluid challenge during the RHC can be helpful to unmask HFpEF in those patients with PAWP ≤ 15 mmHg at rest, even if there is no consensus on the definition for exercise-induced PH or a standardized fluid challenge protocol yet [1].

Table 9.2 Current hemodynamic classification of pulmonary hypertension

Group according to the 5th Word Symposium on pulmonary hypertension	Hemodynamic definition
1. PAH	mPAP≥25 mmHg PAWP≤15 mmHg PVR>3 WU
2. PH due to left heart disease	mPAP≥25 mmHg PAWP>15 mmHg Isolated postcapillary PH: DPD<7 mmHg Combined post-/precapillary PH: DPD≥7 mmHg
3. PH due to lung disease	mPAP≥25 mmHg PAWP≤15 mmHg Severe PH: mPAP≥35 mmHg or mPAP≥25 mmHg and CI<2.0 l/min/m^2
4. Chronic thromboembolic PH	mPAP≥25 mmHg PAWP≤15 mmHg (mPAP<25 mmHg: chronic thromboembolic disease without PH)

Modified from Refs. [1, 19–22]
CI cardiac index, *DPD* diastolic pressure difference (i.e., diastolic pulmonary artery pressure – PAWP), *mPAP* mean pulmonary artery pressure, *PAH* pulmonary arterial hypertension, *PAWP* pulmonary artery wedge pressure, *PH* pulmonary hypertension, *PVR* pulmonary vascular resistance

Many terms have been used to describe the finding of considerably elevated mPAP and PVR in patients with left heart disease and elevated PAWP, for example "out-of-proportion" vs. "proportional" or "reactive" vs. "passive" PH [8, 19]. However, those terms have variable definitions, are based rather on consensus than on evidence, and might have led to an inappropriate use of targeted PAH drugs. The currently proposed definition (see Table 9.2) is based on the diastolic pressure difference (i.e., the difference between diastolic pulmonary artery pressure and PAWP; DPD) instead of the so-called transpulmonary gradient (i.e., the difference between mPAP and PAWP) or PVR, because the diastolic PAP is less influenced by the level of PAWP, cardiac output, and stroke volume compared to the mPAP [23]. Therefore, an elevated DPD may better reflect a relevant pulmonary vascular remodeling than the level of PVR. In normal subjects, DPD ranges between 1 and 3 mmHg. In patients with left heart disease, DPD>5 mmHg was found in about half of patients with PVR>2.5 WU and is discussed to be a marker of "changes in the pulmonary circulation" [19]. An elevation of DPD≥7 mmHg in patients with PH group 2 carried a dismal prognosis similar to PAH in a recent large retrospective study [24]. Therefore it is suggested to differentiate between isolated postcapillary PH (PAWP>15 and DPD<7 mmHg) and combined post-/precapillary PH (PAWP>15 mmHg and DPD≥7 mmHg) [19]. Of note, this definition has no therapeutic implications (vide infra), and it is of utmost importance to exclude relevant lung disease and/or chronic thromboembolic disease in patients with post-/precapillary PH due to left heart diseases.

When PH is present in patients with left heart disease, these have more severe symptoms, worse exercise tolerance, and a worse prognosis [19]. Outcome deteriorates further when right ventricular failure develops [25]. The true prevalence and incidence of PH group 2 is difficult to estimate, because available studies use different definitions of PH, different diagnostic tools (echocardiography or RHC), and examine different populations (e.g., transplant candidates, symptomatic patients, or random samples from the general population). However, because of the high frequency of left heart diseases per se, it is estimated to be the largest PH group by far [26]. As many underlying left heart diseases are more prevalent with increasing age, PH in this group can be also expected to be more prevalent in elderly patients.

Group 3, Pulmonary Hypertension Due to Lung Disease

PH can occur in advanced chronic lung diseases like chronic obstructive pulmonary disease (COPD) and idiopathic pulmonary fibrosis (IPF), but is also found in patients with hypoxia due to sleep apnea or hypoventilation disorders (Table 9.1). On RHC, PH group 3 is typically precapillary (see Table 9.4), even if post-/precapillary PH may occur in patients with lung disease and concomitant left heart disease. With respect to hemodynamic disease severity, there is usually a clear relationship with the underlying lung disease [20, 27, 28]. Importantly, the severity of the lung disease may be underestimated by spirometry, for example in patients with combined pulmonary fibrosis and emphysema who can have virtually normal lung volumes and flows [29]. In patients with only mild lung disease but severe PH, there are usually additional reasons for PH like chronic thromboembolism [30]. In addition, there are very few patients with lung disease and more severe PH, who have to be regarded separately [20]. In the past, these patients with less severe lung disease and more severe PH have been described to have PH "out-of-proportion" [31]. Recently, it has been suggested to use a more descriptive terminology (see Table 9.4), as it is indeed unknown what is "in proportion". It is recommended to distinguish patients with lung disease and no PH (mPAP $<$ 25 mmHg) from those with PH at rest [20]. Patients with mPAP $\geq$ 35 mmHg at rest or mPAP $\geq$ 25 mmHg together with a cardiac index <2.0 l/min/m^2 are described to have "severe group 3 PH". In this group, the differential diagnosis of PAH and concomitant (but not causal) lung disease can be challenging [20, 32].

Although the exact prevalence of group 3 PH is unknown, it is common in advanced stages of COPD and IPF [27, 28]. In patients evaluated for lung transplantation, PH (defined by mPAP $\geq$ 25 mmHg on RHC at rest) was present in about one third of patients and associated with a worse transplant-free survival [33]. Especially in patients with only mildly elevated mPAP it is unclear if PH plays a causal role with respect to prognostic impairment, or if it just reflects the severity for the underlying lung disease. PH due to lung diseases can be expected to be very frequent in elderly patients due to the following reasons. The prevalence of COPD and IPF increases with age [34, 35]. Prevalence and severity of PH increase with duration of the lung disease [36]. Thereby the prevalence of PH in elderly patients with lung diseases may be underestimated as these have not been systematically investigated by RHC (because treatment options which require invasive examination like lung transplantation are age-restricted).

Group 4, Chronic Thromboembolic Pulmonary Hypertension

Chronic thromboembolic PH (CTEPH) can develop after one or more symptomatic venous thromboembolic events, but may also be diagnosed in patients without the history of such an index event [37]. In the absence of left heart disease, CTEPH presents with a precapillary PH (Table 9.2). However, chronic thromboembolic disease can also be responsible for severe symptoms in patients with mPAP < 25 mmHg at rest [21, 38].

The reported cumulative incidence of CTEPH following a symptomatic pulmonary embolism ranges from 0.6 to 3.8 % [39, 40]. As about 25 % of patients with the expert diagnosis of CTEPH in a current registry had no history of pulmonary embolism, the prevalence can be assumed to be even higher [37]. Patients with CTEPH and an mPAP at the time of diagnostic RHC > 30 mmHg at rest who are only treated with therapeutic anticoagulation are reported to have a very poor prognosis with only about 10 % surviving 3 years of follow-up [41]. With the advancement of surgical and anesthesiological techniques, the so-called pulmonary endarterectomy (PEA) has been developed in San Diego, California, which has led to a considerable improvement of outcome over time [42]. Currently, 93 % of operable patients are alive 1 year after the procedure with an in-hospital mortality of 4.7 % [43]. Even if there are no comparative studies, the prognosis of inoperable CTEPH patients did also improve over the recent years, presumably due to (off-label) use of targeted PAH therapy [44].

Because age is a known risk factor for venous thromboembolic events, CTEPH is a common cause of PH in elderly patients. In a current registry of 679 consecutive patients diagnosed with CTEPH between 2/2007 and 1/2009, the median age was 63 years with 25 % of patients being older than 72 years [37]. The rate of comorbidities in these patients was lower than expected with 10 % suffering from COPD and only 2 % of reported left ventricular diastolic dysfunction. In the face of such a positive selection it can be assumed that many elderly patients with CTEPH and more comorbidity are not being sent to expert centers.

Diagnosis and Differential Diagnosis of Pulmonary Hypertension

Symptoms and Clinical Signs

There are no characteristic or even "diagnostic" symptoms reported by patients with PH. In patients with PAH, the most common symptoms dyspnea, fatigue, angina and pre-syncope are graded according to the so-called modified WHO FC from I to IV [8]. Patients with other etiologies of PH may report additional symptoms reflecting the underlying disease such as chronic cough in COPD. The mean time from the onset of symptoms to the diagnostic RHC in patients with PAH is still considerable with 2.8 years in a current registry, which can probably be explained by the unspecific nature and gradual onset of symptoms in PAH [13]. In early stages of PH, there are no typical clinical signs. Distension of the jugular veins, hepatomegaly, peripheral edema, and a split second heart sound can be detected in advanced disease stages or rather in manifest right heart decompensation [8]. Other clinical findings like inspiratory crackles or chronic venous insufficiency can point towards underlying diseases.

It has not been investigated if elderly patients with PH report different symptoms or a different time course of symptom development compared to younger patients. However, elderly PAH patients are more symptomatic at diagnosis compared to younger patients as reflected by a higher mean WHO FC [14, 15]. In addition, at the time of diagnosis elderly patients with PAH more frequently show peripheral edema and report a lower incidence of syncope or pre-syncope until diagnosis [14]. While an analysis from REVEAL found an age <36 years to be the major risk factor for a delayed PAH diagnosis, others reported a significantly longer median duration of 24 months from symptom onset to diagnosis in patients over the age of 50 compared to 12 months in younger patients [14, 45]. The higher number of comorbidities in elderly patients might account for these observations. In REVEAL, a history of obstructive airway disease and sleep apnea were also independently associated with delayed PAH recognition [45]. Another reason might be that older patients (and maybe their relatives) explain their symptoms by aging itself and seek medical help later in the course of the disease accordingly.

Echocardiography

When PH is clinically suspected, echocardiography is the screening method of choice [8]. Current guidelines focus on the systolic PAP and suggest arbitrary cutoff values to estimate the likelihood for PH (e.g. PH is "unlikely" with systolic PAP$\leq$36 mmHg) [8]. As PAP estimation on echocardiography is often inaccurate or impossible (in patients without insufficiency of the tricuspid valve), other signs like dilatation of the right heart chambers should be considered [46–48]. This may be especially important in elderly PAH patients who show lower mean PAP values on diagnosis compared to younger patients [15].

In addition to estimation of the likelihood for PH, echocardiography is important with respect to differential diagnosis. Left ventricular function (systolic and diastolic) and left sided valve diseases can be assessed and related to the severity of PH. The presence of congenital heart diseases such as atrial septal defects or a partial anomalous pulmonary venous connection should also be considered in elderly patients presenting with PH. A comprehensive echocardiographic evaluation including transesophageal studies could prevent underdiagnosis. On the other hand, it can be difficult (if not impossible) to reliably establish or exclude a causal relationship between a left heart abnormality and PH [19]. This may be even more challenging in elderly patients with PH due to the high prevalence of left heart diseases.

Thoracic Imaging

PH can be suspected on chest X-ray, which is abnormal in the majority of patients with PAH at diagnosis [12]. On chest computed tomography (CT), a dilatation of the pulmonary artery trunk can indicate PH [49]. However, the pulmonary artery diameter is also increasing with age in normal subjects and should therefore be used cautiously to predict PH [50].

The main indication for thoracic imaging studies in patients with (suspected) PH is differential diagnosis. A high-resolution CT scan of the chest can detect pronounced abnormalities of the lung parenchyma even in the absence of a relevant impairment on spirometry, for example in patients with combined pulmonary fibrosis and emphysema [29]. Further, it is important in the differential diagnosis of pulmonary veno-occlusive disease [8]. When intravenous contrast can be administered (regarding kidney and thyroid function), chronic thromboembolic disease can also be detected [51]. Of note, signs of chronic thromboembolism are very different from those of an acute pulmonary embolism and can easily be missed. In addition to particularly looking for webs, bands, thrombus calcifications, bronchial artery hypertrophy (requiring contrast medium also in the aorta), sudden changes in vessel caliber, poststenotic dilatation, and mosaic perfusion, the use of reconstructions with thin sections ($\leq$1 mm) can be helpful for detection [22]. Importantly, a chest CT scan should not be used for exclusion of chronic thromboembolic disease except at very experienced centers [8].

In general, a ventilation/perfusion (V/Q) scan by nuclear imaging has a high sensitivity for the detection of acute and chronic pulmonary embolism which present with similar signs [52, 53]. The sensitivity can be further improved by using single photon emission CT (SPECT) technique, which should be the standard test to rule out chronic thromboembolism in patients with PH [22]. However, especially in patients with inhomogeneous distribution of the inhaled radiopharmakon as for example in severe COPD, the number of non-diagnostic V/Q scans increases [54]. With advancement of CT techniques like dual-energy CT for the assessment of pulmonary perfusion, V/Q scans might become less important in the future [55].

Due to the wide availability and the high diagnostic yield of CT, direct pulmonary angiography is nowadays rarely used in the diagnosis of acute pulmonary embolism. However, angiography is still the gold standard for diagnosis of chronic thromboembolic disease and for operability assessment in many PEA expert centers [22]. It could be combined with the diagnostic RHC to increase patient comfort and the quality of angiographic images (due to adaption of the contrast medium flow rate to cardiac output). Although thoracic/cardiac magnetic resonance imaging (MRI) has the capability to non-invasively assess PAP, left and right ventricular function, cardiac output, shunts, and pulmonary perfusion, its use is currently limited to special clinical questions and research due to availability and costs [56].

Right Heart Catheterization

The gold standard of PH diagnosis is RHC [1]. In addition, it is needed for differentiation between pre- and postcapillary PH, for assessment of PH severity, and for exclusion of left-to-right shunts. Following the 5th World Symposium on PH in 2013, consensus recommendations have been made for RHC measurements which can influence levels of mPAP and PAWP (in addition to age) [1]. The zero level of the pressure transducer should be set at the half of the anterior-posterior thoracic diameter which reflects the level of the left atrium [57]. According to respiratory swings of the pressure curves, endexpiratory values should be recorded rather than digital means to avoid an overdiagnosis of precapillary PH. Pressure values in the right atrium, right ventricle, pulmonary artery (systolic, diastolic), and in the "wedge" position should be measured repeatedly (especially PAWP) and documented on every RHC report. Further it is essential to measure cardiac output by either the direct Fick method or thermodilution for calculation of PVR, and to assess the mixed venous oxygen saturation to not miss a relevant left-to-right shunt [1]. The testing of vasoreactivity is only indicated in patients with idiopathic PAH to identify possible calcium channel blocker (CCB) responders (see section "Pulmonary arterial hypertension"). Patients with other etiologies of PAH and PH should not be routinely tested as a positive test result may occur, but CCB therapy can be ineffective or even harmful [58]. Therefore, the non-invasive differential diagnostic tests should usually be done before proceeding to RHC. Furthermore, patients with clinical signs of cardiac failure should preferably be catheterized after re-compensation first, because otherwise high cardiac filling pressures may lead to overestimation of pulmonary pressures and the hemodynamic finding of post-/precapillary PH with consecutive diagnostic uncertainty and the need for repeat RHC.

Algorithm of Differential Diagnosis

The currently suggested algorithm for the differential diagnostic assessment of patients with suspected PH is given in Fig. 9.1. If all mentioned investigations are adequately performed, it should be possible to allocate the patient to one out of five groups of the PH classifications system accordingly (Table 9.1). However, the complexity of differential diagnosis increases with age and the number of comorbidities, especially if these can also cause PH.

With respect to idiopathic PAH, we have a "classical" phenotype in mind, which is best reflected by the historical data from the NIH registry [12]. Patients with PPH showed a female preponderance, a mean age of 36 years, a very severe PH on RHC, and virtually no comorbidities. Of note, the inclusion criteria and mandatory investigations for exclusion of "secondary" PH forms were very strict at that time (e.g. normal V/Q scan or pulmonary angiography mandatory to exclude CTEPH).

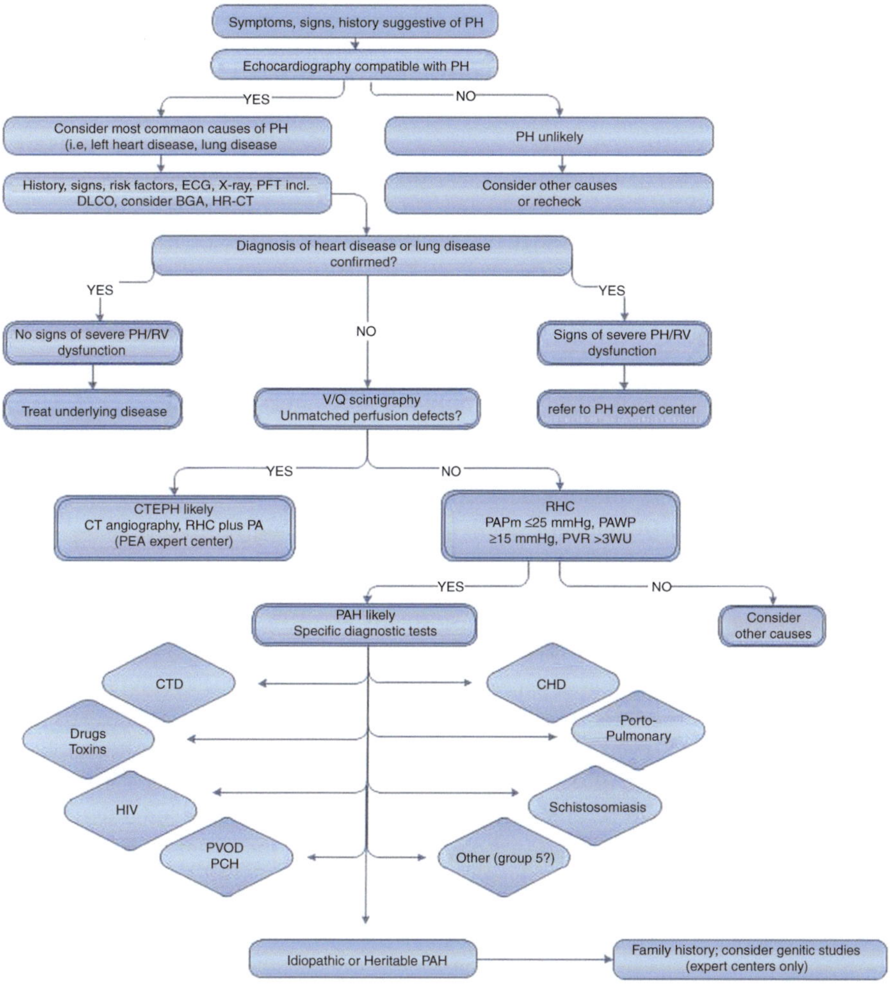

Fig. 9.1 Diagnostic approach to patients with suspected pulmonary hypertension. *BGA* blood gas analysis, *CHD* congenital heart disease, *CTD* connective tissue disease, *CTEPH* chronic thromboembolic pulmonary hypertension, *DLCO* diffusion capacity of the lung for carbon monoxide, *ECG* electrocardiogram, *HR-CT* high-resolution computed tomography, *PA* pulmonary angiography, *PAH* pulmonary arterial hypertension, *PAPm* mean pulmonary artery pressure, *PAWP* pulmonary arterial wedge pressure, *PCH* pulmonary capillary hemangiomatosis, *PEA* pulmonary endarterectomy, *PFT* pulmonary function testing, *PH* pulmonary hypertension, *PVOD* pulmonary veno-occlusive disease, *PVR* pulmonary vascular resistance, *RHC* right heart catheter, *RV* right ventricle, *V/Q* ventilation/perfusion, *x-ray* chest radiograph (From Ref. [1])

However, age ranged from 1 to 81 years, and 9 % of PPH patients were older than 60 years, indicating that age alone cannot be used to exclude a diagnosis of idiopathic PAH. In addition, the mean age of patients with PAH associated with connective tissue disease is usually higher compared to idiopathic PAH [13].

There are no data directly comparing hemodynamic disease severity in elderly patients diagnosed with idiopathic PAH at the time of the NIH registry and today. However, with increasing mean age we observe lower mean mPAP, higher mean PAWP, and lower PVR compared to patient populations with a lower mean age (NIH registry, Chinese registry). A current analysis from COMPERA even found a significant inverse relationship between age and mPAP on PAH diagnosis, suggesting a worse capability of the "older" right ventricle to adapt to increased PVR [15]. The higher mean PAWP can be explained by the age-dependent increase in left ventricular filling pressures even in normal subjects [59]. The REVEAL registry included patients with slightly elevated PAWP at rest (16–18 mmHg), who otherwise showed hemodynamic characteristics typical for PAH (severely elevated mean mPAP above 50 mmHg, decreased cardiac index, very high PVR), and in whom alternative causes for PH (e.g., relevant lung disease or chronic thromboembolic disease) were excluded [17]. These patients received an "expert diagnosis" of PAH and treatment with targeted PAH therapy accordingly. Compared to PAH patients with PAWP $\leq$ 15 mmHg at rest, they were significantly older, more obese, and had more comorbidities associated with left heart disease, but showed a similar survival on targeted PAH therapy.

A major challenge in (elderly) patients with lung diseases (e.g., COPD, IPF), history of venous thromboembolism or even signs of chronic thromboembolic disease on CT or V/Q scan, and left heart diseases (especially HFpEF) is to establish or exclude a causal relationship between PH severity and the underlying disease. While this seems to be clear for example in patients with advanced lung diseases and non-severe PH (Table 9.2), the situation is less evident in patients with mild lung disease (e.g. COPD GOLD II) and severe PH [20, 31]. After exclusion of chronic thromboembolic disease and abnormalities of the lung parenchyma on high-resolution CT scan of the chest, such a patient may be diagnosed with PAH and concomitant lung disease and treated accordingly. To avoid an overdiagnosis of PAH, the differential diagnostic assessment should be very thorough and preferably be performed at experienced centers [8, 20]. Similar considerations may occur in patients with HFpEF and a normal PAWP at rest but severely elevated mPAP and PVR, or in patients with minor findings of chronic thromboembolic disease on chest CT but normal V/Q scan. In addition, patients with definitive signs of chronic thromboembolic disease can sometimes turn out to have clear postcapillary PH on RHC, which should prompt further diagnosis and therapy of left heart disease instead of proceeding to PEA. Further, patients with chronic thromboembolic disease may have normal mPAP at rest, but dyspnea due to V/Q mismatch or PH on exercise [21].

Up to date there is no consensus on criteria for allocation of patients with PH and left heart or lung diseases to the groups 1, 2, or 3 of the PH classification system depending on severity of PH and the underlying disease. However, with a thorough differential diagnostic assessment and application of strict criteria for the diagnosis of PAH, the majority of elderly PH patients presenting to PH expert centers will receive an alternative diagnosis [60]. It should be in our interest to conduct prospective clinical trials in the (often elderly) patients with "relevant" underlying left heart or lung diseases and more severe PH to assess the efficacy and safety of currently available targeted PAH therapy.

Therapy of Pulmonary Hypertension

In the treatment algorithm for PAH, general measures and supportive therapy are recommended according to available evidence (Fig. 9.2) [61]. In part, these recommendations also apply for other forms of PH. Supervised exercise training is an established part of therapy in patients with left heart failure and pulmonary diseases and should also be prescribed when PH (group 2 or 3) is complicating the underlying disease. The absolute measurable effect of exercise training may be less pronounced in elderly patients. However, also seemingly small effects can be valuable for the individual patient, and age should not be a reason to withhold prescription of a supervised training program. Importantly patients should be clinically stable and optimally treated for underlying diseases and PH [62]. Even if in patients with PH due to left heart and lung diseases, strenuous physical activity may be less harmful compared to patients with severe idiopathic PAH or CTEPH, it should be avoided. Other recommendations made on the basis of expert consensus include immunizations and the avoidance of pregnancy. Diuretics and fluid restriction are part of the basic treatment of heart failure in general, oxygen therapy should be prescribed according to separate guidelines. Therapeutic anticoagulation is recommended for patients with idiopathic, heritable and anorexigen-associated PAH and mandatory in CTEPH [22, 61]. In other PH groups, anticoagulation is not generally recommended and should only be prescribed if other indications like atrial fibrillation are present.

Pulmonary Arterial Hypertension

In the current PAH treatment algorithm as shown in Fig. 9.2, specific age groups are not considered, although there are specific recommendations for pediatric patients [63]. General measures and supportive therapy as described above should be applicable for elderly PAH patients, too. The same applies for supervised exercise training, which has not yet been analyzed with respect to age-dependent effects, but the majority of studies also included elderly patients [62]. Therapeutic anticoagulation is only recommended for idiopathic, heritable and anorexigen-associated PAH on the basis of historical data [8]. In the so far largest (retrospective) analysis showing a survival benefit with therapeutic anticoagulation in patients with idiopathic PAH (n = 800; 66 % received anticoagulation) in the modern treatment era, the median age was 70 years [64]. Therefore, therapeutic anticoagulation can also be recommended in elderly patients in these specific PAH subgroups. Of note, because there are no data on newer oral anticoagulants in PAH patients, vitamin K antagonists are still recommended as treatment of choice [61].

Vasoreactivity testing for identification of CCB responders should only be performed in patients with idiopathic PAH as other PAH subgroups rarely respond to CCB therapy even after an acute positive testing result (defined as a reduction of mPAP $\geq$ 10 mmHg to reach an absolute value of mPAP $\leq$ 40 with an increased or unchanged cardiac output [65]) [1, 58]. There is no clear relationship between age

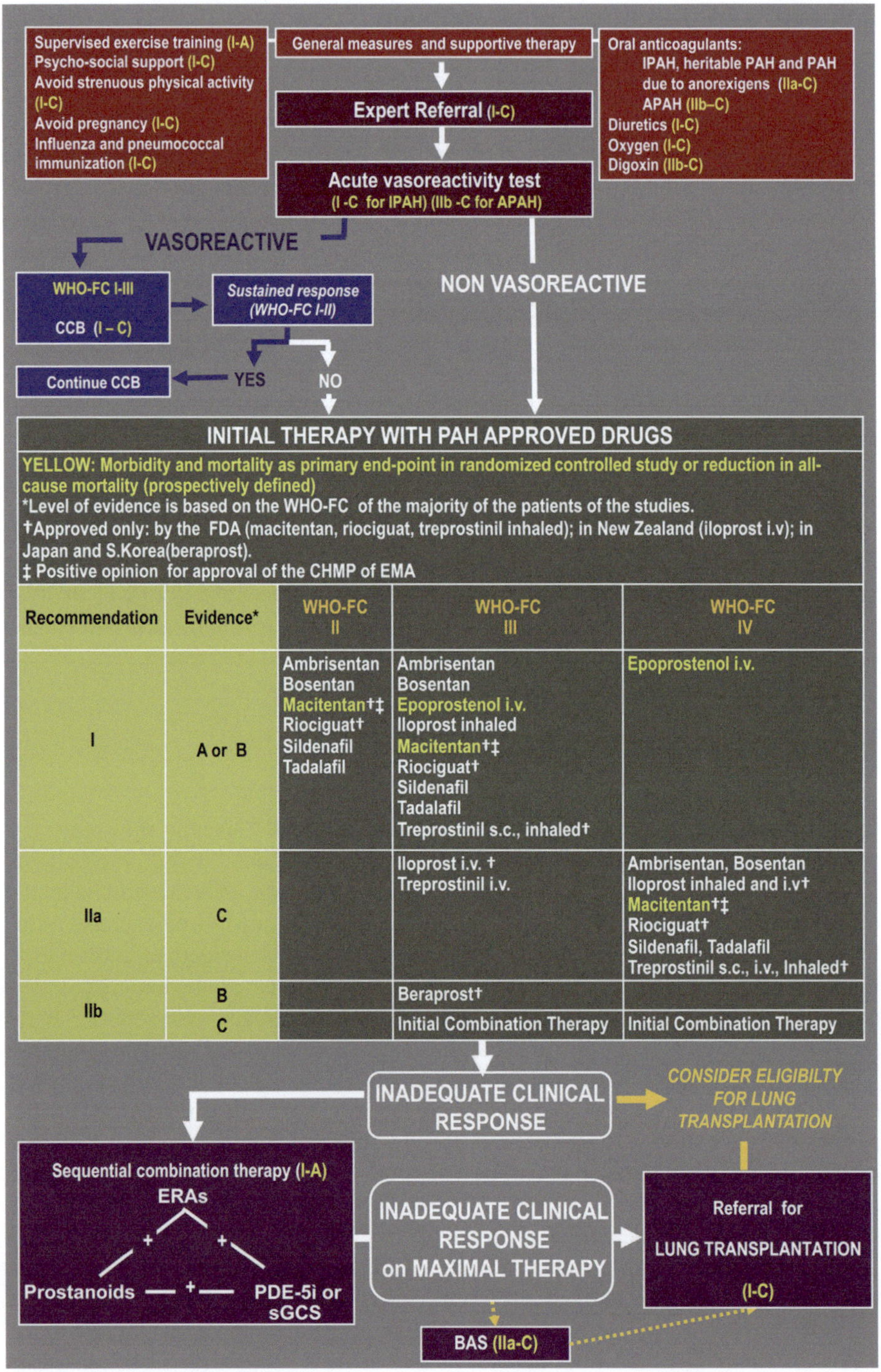

Fig. 9.2 Treatment algorithm of pulmonary arterial hypertension. *APAH* associated pulmonary arterial hypertension, *BAS* balloon atrial septostomy, *CCB* calcium channel blockers, *ERA* endothelin receptor antagonist, *sGCS* soluble guanylate cyclase stimulators, *IPAH* idiopathic pulmonary arterial hypertension, *i.v.* intravenous, *PDE-5i* phosphodiesterase type-5 inhibitor, *s.c.* subcutaneous, *WHO-FC* World Health Organization functional class (From Ref. [61])

and vasoreactivity [65, 66], although some studies found that responders were younger compared to non-responders [67]. However, every patient with suspected idiopathic PAH should be tested regardless of age, and patients with a positive test should be treated with CCB as long as they are in a good WHO FC [61]. Possible substances for vasoreactivity testing are inhaled nitric oxide (10–20 ppm), intravenous Epoprostenol (2–12 ng/kg/min) or Adenosine (50–350 mg/min), and inhaled Iloprost (5 μg) [1].

The so-called "targeted PAH therapy," consisting of endothelin receptor antagonists (ERA), phosphodiesterase 5-inhibitors (PDE 5-I), prostaglandin analogs, and Riociguat, is licensed for the treatment of PAH without age-restrictions [61]. The current standard of care is initiation of monotherapy according to published evidence and WHO FC as displayed in Fig. 9.2, followed by sequential addition of another targeted PAH agent if treatment goals are not met. This concept (sequential additive therapy with Bosentan, Sildenafil, Iloprost, and lung transplantation) has been evaluated in comparison with a historical control group (only therapy with prostaglandin analogs and lung transplantation available) of similar age and hemodynamic disease severity, and showed a significantly improved outcome [68]. Newer studies of sequential or initial combination therapy support an even earlier treatment with at least two targeted PAH drugs to improve the further course of the disease also in apparently stable PAH patients [69, 70]. However, these new data, which are in part only available in abstract form to date, have not led to a change of recommendations yet.

Currently recommended treatment goals are displayed in Table 9.3 [71]. The given cutoff values are chosen arbitrarily from different clinical studies and do not consider age in particular. Of course, most of the mentioned parameters are clearly age-dependent, for example cardiac output and exercise capacity. Therefore, clinicians presumably apply a kind of "physiologic age-correction," for example in the assessment of WHO FC (i.e. expecting a certain level of dyspnea for a certain level of exercise which is lower for elderly patients). However, this approach, although most likely practiced, is apparently very subjective. For WHO FC, this could perhaps be improved by the use of standardized questionnaires. For biomarkers like NT pro-BNP, the upper limit of normal is increasing with age and reported accordingly by the laboratory. A possible way to correct for the physiologic age-related decrease in exercise capacity could be the use of % predicted instead of absolute values when suitable equations are available. For example, % predicted of peak oxygen uptake on cardiopulmonary exercise testing at baseline better predicted long-term survival in 226 patients with idiopathic and heritable PAH compared to absolute values (using $ml*kg^{-1}*min^{-1}$) [72]. Elderly PAH patients show shorter distances on the standardized 6 min walk test, and less often achieve thresholds known to be associated with an improved prognosis on therapy [15, 73]. In a retrospective study, elderly patients on targeted PAH therapy were more likely to reach a threshold of 78 % predicted 6 min walk distance instead of the corresponding absolute value of 380 m, while the usefulness of prognostication was not affected [73]. Therefore, such corrections could be useful in daily clinical practice to avoid over- or under-treatment of elderly patients.

Table 9.3 Variables used in clinical practice to determine response to therapy and prognosis in patients with PAH

Variable	Target range
WHO functional class	I or II
Echocardiography/cardiac magnetic resonance imaging	Normal/near-normal RV size and function
Hemodynamics	Normalization of RV function ($RAP < 8$ mmHg and $CI > 2.5$ to 3.0 l/min/m^2)
6-min walk distance	>380–440 m; may not be aggressive enough in young individuals
Cardiopulmonary exercise testing	Peak-$VO_2 > 15$ ml/min/kg and $EqCO_2 < 45$
B-type natriuretic peptide level	Normal

Modified from Ref. [71]

CI cardiac index, *$EqCO_2$* ventilatory equivalent for carbon dioxide, *PAH* pulmonary arterial hypertension, *RAP* right atrial pressure, *RV* right ventricular, *VO_2* peak oxygen consumption

Elderly PAH patients show higher WHO FC and lower 6 min walk distances both at diagnosis and on targeted therapy [15]. According to the "treat-to-target" concept recommended in current guidelines, they should theoretically receive an even higher amount of combination therapy (2 or 3 targeted PAH drugs) compared to younger patients. However, elderly patients less often receive combination therapy, prostaglandin analogs, and lung transplantation in the real world [14]. While the latter can be explained by age-restrictions for transplantation, the reasons for the remaining observations are less evident. Worse tolerance of some targeted PAH medications could play a role as indicated by a higher discontinuation rate of ERA in elderly PAH patients [15]. In addition, the complexity of application (especially parenteral therapy with prostaglandin analogs) and the considerable costs of therapy may play a role.

It is unclear if the worse survival observed in elderly PAH patients can be explained by the restrictive use of combination therapy and if outcome, exercise capacity, and quality of life could be improved by application of more aggressive treatment strategies. However, especially in elderly PAH patients individual treatment goals should be set in agreement with the respective patient, taking into account comorbidities, side effects of therapy, individual patient preferences, and the "biologic" rather than the "numeric" age. Of course, age alone should not be regarded a contraindication for combination therapy or more invasive treatments like application of parenteral prostaglandin analogs.

Pulmonary Hypertension in Left Heart Diseases

There are no specific recommendations for the treatment of PH in patients with left heart disease except treating the underlying condition [8]. In particular, patients with group 2 PH should not be treated with targeted PAH drugs, because controlled clinical trials so far have shown no benefit or even harm [8, 19, 74]. However, these trials usually mixed up patients with isolated postcapillary PH and patients with a

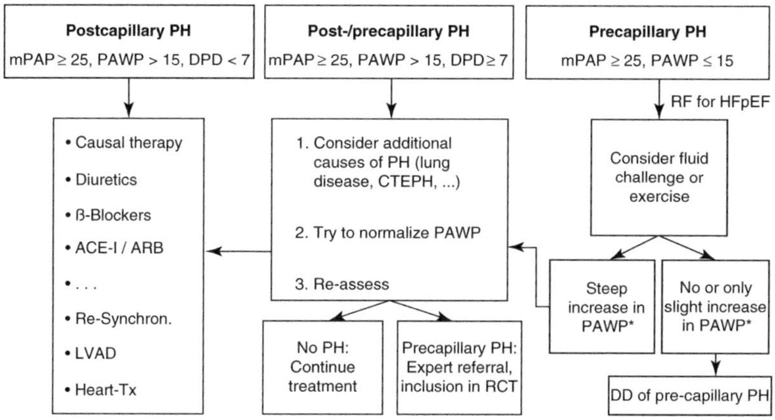

Fig. 9.3 Proposed algorithm for diagnosis and therapy in pulmonary hypertension due to left heart disease. *currently not defined by consensus, *ACE*-I angiotensin converting enzyme inhibitors, *ARB* angiotensin receptor blockers, *CTEPH* chronic thromboembolic pulmonary hypertension, *DD* differential diagnosis, *DPD* diastolic pressure difference (i.e., diastolic pulmonary artery pressure – PAWP), *HFpEF* heart failure with preserved ejection fraction, *LVAD* left ventricular assist device, *mPAP* mean pulmonary artery pressure, *PAWP* pulmonary artery wedge pressure, *PH* pulmonary hypertension, *RCT* randomized controlled trial, *Re-Synchron.* resynchronization therapy (i.e., by means of biventricular pacemaker stimulation), *Tx* transplantation

"precapillary component" of their PH (now defined as post-/precapillary PH, see Table 9.2), who should be regarded separately. With successful treatment of the underlying left heart disease according to current guidelines, including "aggressive" drug therapy, operative or interventional therapy of mitral and aortic valve disease, device therapy, and finally heart transplantation, PH should be reversible in patients with isolated postcapillary PH (see Fig. 9.3).

In patients with post-/precapillary PH it may be hard to accept the causal role of the left heart disease, especially if mPAP is elevated to above 40 or 50 mmHg. However, even if tempting, these patients should not directly be diagnosed with PAH and treated accordingly, because pulmonary vasodilatation by targeted PAH drugs can lead to pulmonary edema and deterioration of left heart disease [8, 19]. So first, additional reasons for precapillary PH should be accurately excluded, because lung diseases and chronic thromboembolic disease are common in elderly patients and share risk factors with cardiovascular diseases like cigarette smoking. Second, the underlying left heart disease should be adequately treated (Fig. 9.3). If either post-/precapillary PH or even precapillary PH persists on re-evaluation (usually after 3–6 months), there is a potential rationale for the use of targeted PAH drugs [19]. In some patients it may then even be difficult to differentiate between PAH and PH group 2 with extensive pulmonary vascular remodeling. However, given the rarity of "classic" IPAH in elderly patients [60], targeted PAH therapy should be prescribed with caution and by dedicated expert centers only. In addition, patients with group 2 post-/precapillary PH as described should be candidates for randomized clinical trials utilizing targeted PAH therapy [19].

In patients with precapillary PH at rest but risk factors for or echocardiographic signs of HFpEF, a fluid challenge or slight exercise on RHC should be considered especially when mPAP and PVR are only slightly elevated [1]. When a steep increase in PAWP is observed, patients should be treated according to guidelines for left heart disease, even if there is no drug therapy of proven benefit for HFpEF so far. Although PDE 5-I have shown promise in selected patients with severe HFpEF and PH, larger studies failed to show a beneficial effect [75, 76]. Therefore, especially patients with HFpEF and mild PH should not be treated with any targeted PAH therapy. In patients with normal PAWP at rest, "mild" signs of HFpEF and more severe PH, the whole spectrum of differential diagnoses of precapillary PH including PAH should be considered. Patients with suspected PAH and concomitant HFpEF should be referred to a PAH expert center for further diagnostic evaluation, initiation of targeted therapy, and follow-up.

Pulmonary Hypertension in Lung Diseases

In patients with PH due to lung diseases, current guidelines focus on the treatment of the underlying disease [8]. This comprises oxygen therapy in patients with hypoxemia, inhalation of bronchodilators in COPD, immunosuppression in some interstitial lung diseases, non-invasive ventilation in sleep apnea and hypoventilation disorders, and finally lung transplantation in suitable patients. For some of these therapies, a considerable positive effect on the severity of PH is described, for example that of effective non-invasive ventilation in patients with PH due to obesity hypoventilation syndrome [77]. On the other hand, even measures known to prolong survival like long-term oxygen therapy in COPD, have only a marginal effect on hemodynamics in these patients [78].

As patients with lung diseases show worse exercise capacity and survival when PH develops [27, 33, 79], effects of targeted PAH therapy have also been investigated. In summary, studies on acute hemodynamics and small uncontrolled series often showed positive effects, while randomized placebo-controlled trials looking for an improvement in exercise capacity were negative so far [80–82]. Possible explanations for the failure of PAH targeted therapy to significantly improve exercise capacity in patients with PH and lung diseases include V/Q mismatch, which can be exaggerated by PAH drugs, and hypoxemia due to the lung disease itself which is commonly not influenced by PAH targeted therapy but limits exercise capacity [83]. In addition, the majority of studies included patients with advanced lung disease but only mild PH, and some diagnosed PH by echocardiography only. It might be possible that targeted PAH therapy prolongs survival even in the absence of exercise capacity improvement [32]. However, prospective controlled studies are needed to test this hypothesis. Currently, the use of targeted PAH therapy is not recommended in patients with group 3 PH [8].

A minority of patients with lung diseases shows severe PH on RHC (Table 9.2). If other conditions potentially influencing PH severity like chronic

Table 9.4 Differential diagnosis between PAH (group 1) and PH due to lung diseases (group 3)

Criteria favoring PAH (group 1)	Parameter	Criteria favoring PH due to lung disease (group 3)
Normal or mildly impaired $FEV_1 > 60$ % pred. (COPD) $FVC > 70$ % pred. (IPF)	Ventilatory function/spirometry	Moderate to severe impairment $FEV_1 < 60$ % pred. (COPD) $FVC < 70$ % pred. (IPF)
Absence or only "modest" airway or parenchymal abnormalities	High-resolution CT scan[a]	Characteristic airway and/or parenchymal abnormalities
Features of exhausted circulatory reserve[b] Preserved breathing reserve Reduced oxygen pulse Low CO/VO_2-slope SvO_2 at lower limit No change or decrease in $PaCO_2$ during exercise	Cardiopulmonary exercise testing (including hemodynamics)	Features of exhausted ventilatory reserve Reduced breathing reserve Normal oxygen pulse Normal CO/VO_2-slope SvO_2 above lower limit Increase in $PaCO_2$ during exercise

Modified from Ref. [20]

CO/VO_2 cardiac output/oxygen consumption ratio, *COPD* chronic obstructive pulmonary disease, *CT* computed tomography, *DPLD* diffuse parenchymal lung disease, *FEV_1* forced expiratory volume in first second, *FVC* forced vital capacity, *IPF* idiopathic pulmonary fibrosis, *$PaCO_2$* partial pressure of carbon dioxide in arterial blood, *PAH* pulmonary arterial hypertension, *PH* pulmonary hypertension, *PVOD* pulmonary veno-occlusive disease, *SvO_2* mixed venous oxygen saturation

[a]As to CT diagnosis, parenchymal changes linked to PVOD are to be discriminated from those associated with DPLD

[b]Features of exhausted circulatory reserve are also noted in severe PH-COPD and severe PH-IPF, but are then accompanied by major lung function and CT abnormalities

thromboembolic disease are excluded, the two remaining differential diagnoses are severe PH *due* to lung disease and PAH with *concomitant* (usually mild) lung disease [20]. The further assessment and judgment should be performed at experienced PH centers who can also include patients with severe group 3 PH into adequate clinical trials which are urgently needed. The degree of hemodynamic PH severity has to be correlated with the severity of the underlying lung disease, taking into account not only spirometry but also abnormalities on high-resolution CT scans and results of cardiopulmonary exercise testing [20]. An overview of criteria currently suggested for differentiation between PAH and PH due to lung disease is given in Table 9.4. When treating patients with severe PH and relevant lung diseases with targeted PAH therapy (assuming a diagnosis of PAH and concomitant lung disease), a possibly diminished effect on exercise capacity as discussed above has to be taken into account and should also be communicated to the patient. The definition of individual treatment goals in these patients, especially if they are older, is both important and very difficult, as targets applying for "classic" PAH cannot just be transferred to this patient group.

Chronic Thromboembolic Pulmonary Hypertension

The goals in patients with CTEPH are to restore V/Q matching and relieve right heart strain by reduction/normalization of PVR, as both is contributing to dyspnea in a varying proportion [84]. These aims could be ideally accomplished by a complete desobliteration of the pulmonary circulation, while a drug-mediated pulmonary vasodilation can only be expected to lower right ventricular afterload without having marked effects on V/Q mismatch. Due to these pathophysiologic considerations and impressive results regarding functional status and survival, PEA is currently recommended as standard therapy in technically operable CTEPH patients [22]. In a current prospective international registry, 386 (57 %) of 679 consecutive patients with CTEPH underwent PEA in dedicated expert centers [43]. The in-hospital and 1-year mortality was 4.7 % and 7.0 %, respectively, which is clearly better compared to both patients on anticoagulation only (historical data) and on (off-label) treatment with targeted PAH therapy (registry data, mostly inoperable patients) [44]. In patients evaluated 1 year after PEA, the mean PVR decreased from 698 to 235 dyn*s*cm^{-5}, the mean 6-min walk distance increased from 362 to 459 m, and WHO FC improved from III/IV to I/II in the vast majority of patients [43].

The mean age of patients who underwent PEA was 60 years, ranging from 18 to 84 years. Even if patients deemed inoperable were significantly older compared to operable patients (median age 67 vs. 61 years, $p<0.001$), age alone was reported to be the reason for inoperability in only 5 patients (2 %) [37]. The main specific reason was inaccessibility of the occlusions (n = 118; 48 %), followed by comorbidities (n = 33; 13 %) and imbalance between increased PVR and amount of accessible occlusions (i.e. due to pulmonary vascular remodeling) in 25 patients (10 %). Therefore, the age difference between operable and inoperable patients may be partially explained by a higher rate of comorbidities in older patients. In addition, 27 % of inoperable patients had another disease reported, which could be causally linked to PH (compared to 17 % in operable patients; $p=0.002$); and the most frequent diseases (COPD, sleep disorder breathing, left ventricular diastolic dysfunction, left-sided valvular heart disease, and interstitial lung disease) are again age-related. The most frequent reason in technically operable patients not to proceed to PEA was refusal of surgery by the patients (37 of 427; 9 %), which might happen much more frequently in daily clinical practice. Therefore, every patient with a diagnosis of CTEPH should be seen by an experienced PEA team for individual risk stratification and counseling, and age alone should not be regarded a contraindication for surgery especially in otherwise healthy elderly patients [22].

CTEPH does not arise from physical pulmonary artery obstruction alone [84]. In addition, vasoconstriction and pulmonary vascular remodeling can occur on the basis of shear stress and lead to perpetuation and worsening of the disease. The amount and time course of pulmonary vascular remodeling is difficult to predict in individual patients, but it can lead to imbalance between PVR increase and amount of accessible occlusions, higher PEA mortality, and finally inoperability. In addition, remodeling can be a reason for residual PH after PEA. In the situations of surgical inaccessibility or residual PH following PEA, the guanylate cyclase stimulator riociguat has been evaluated in a double-blind, placebo-controlled, randomized study [85]. After 16 weeks of treatment including 8 weeks of up-titration of riociguat, the 6-min walk distance, which was the primary endpoint, increased by a mean of 39 m in the riociguat group, as compared with a mean decrease of 6 m in the placebo group (least-squares mean difference, 46 m; 95 % confidence interval, 25–67; $p<0.001$). In addition, there were significant positive effects on PVR, NT-pro BNP, and WHO FC. Riociguat has consequently been approved for patients with inoperable CTEPH or residual PH after PEA and is now widely available. Even if not yet supported by systemic evidence, the availability of a medication may now increase the awareness for CTEPH, which is currently already seen in clinical practice. Of note, riociguat has not been tested in patients with operable CTEPH (e.g., patients refusing surgery) or inoperability on the basis of comorbidity, and should not be regarded an alternative to PEA. Before initiating riociguat therapy, the diagnosis of CTEPH should be reliably established including imaging and RHC (especially excluding postcapillary PH in elderly patients), and patients should be seen by an experienced PEA team or at least in a PH expert center for risk stratification and counselling [22]. Especially patients with comorbidities of the left heart and/or the lungs should be treated with caution and seen frequently for monitoring of side effects (e.g., pulmonary edema in patients with concomitant left heart disease; worsening of hypoxemia in patients with concomitant COPD or IPF). Further, the effect of riociguat treatment on exercise capacity might be less pronounced in elderly patients with comorbidities compared to the very distinct population included in the pivotal trial.

An additional reason for expert referral of patients with CTEPH is the availability of novel therapeutic methods like pulmonary balloon angioplasty. After having shown a high complication rate initially [86], this technique has been refined by endovascular ultrasound, and recently impressive results with respect to hemodynamic and functional improvement have been reported [87]. Even if there are no studies which compared this procedure to PEA or medical therapy, it is promising especially in patients with surgically inaccessible lesions. From the pathophysiological view, balloon angioplasty should be more effective compared to medical therapy alone, as the V/Q mismatch is also partially restored by the procedure. However, balloon angioplasty should only be performed in experienced PEA centers after comprehensive diagnostic testing and should not be regarded as alternative therapy in operable CTEPH patients.

References

1. Hoeper MM, Bogaard HJ, Condliffe R, et al. Definitions and diagnosis of pulmonary hypertension. J Am Coll Cardiol. 2013;62:D42–50.
2. Kovacs G, Berghold A, Scheidl S, et al. Pulmonary arterial pressure during rest and exercise in healthy subjects: a systematic review. Eur Respir J. 2009;34:888–94.

3. Badesch DB, Champion HC, Gomez Sanchez MA, et al. Diagnosis and assessment of pulmonary arterial hypertension. J Am Coll Cardiol. 2009;54:S55–66.
4. Fujimoto N, Borlaug BA, Lewis GD, et al. Hemodynamic responses to rapid saline loading: the impact of age, sex, and heart failure. Circulation. 2013;127:55–62.
5. Simonneau G, Galiè N, Rubin LJ, et al. Clinical classification of pulmonary hypertension. J Am Coll Cardiol. 2004;43:5S–12.
6. Simonneau G, Gatzoulis MA, Adatia I, et al. Updated clinical classification of pulmonary hypertension. J Am Coll Cardiol. 2013;62:D34–41.
7. Hatano S, Strasser T. Primary pulmonary hypertension. Report on a WHO meeting. Geneva: The WHO; 1975. ISBN 92 4 156044.
8. Galie N, Hoeper MM, Humbert M, et al. Guidelines for the diagnosis and treatment of pulmonary hypertension. The task force for the diagnosis and treatment of pulmonary hypertension of the European Society of Cardiology (ESC) and the European Respiratory Society (ERS), endorsed by the International Society of Heart and Lung Transplantation (ISHLT). Eur Respir J. 2009;34:1219–63.
9. McGoon MD, Benza RL, Escribano-Subias P, et al. Pulmonary arterial hypertension: epidemiology and registries. J Am Coll Cardiol. 2013;62:D51–9.
10. D'Alonzo GE, Barst RJ, Ayres SM, et al. Survival in patients with primary pulmonary hypertension. Results from a national prospective registry. Ann Intern Med. 1991;115:343–9.
11. Benza RL, Miller DP, Barst RJ, et al. An evaluation of long-term survival from time of diagnosis in pulmonary arterial hypertension from the REVEAL Registry. Chest. 2012;142:448–56.
12. Rich S, Dantzker DR, Ayres SM, et al. Primary pulmonary hypertension. A national prospective study. Ann Intern Med. 1987;107:216–23.
13. Badesch DB, Raskob GE, Elliott CG, et al. Pulmonary arterial hypertension: baseline characteristics from the REVEAL Registry. Chest. 2010;137:376–87.
14. Ling Y, Johnson MK, Kiely DG, et al. Changing demographics, epidemiology, and survival of incident pulmonary arterial hypertension: results from the pulmonary hypertension registry of the United Kingdom and Ireland. Am J Respir Crit Care Med. 2012;186:790–6.
15. Hoeper MM, Huscher D, Ghofrani HA, et al. Elderly patients diagnosed with idiopathic pulmonary arterial hypertension: results from the COMPERA registry. Int J Cardiol. 2013;168: 871–80.
16. Zhang R, Dai L, Xie W, et al. Survival of Chinese patients with pulmonary arterial hypertension in the modern treatment era. Chest. 2011;140:301–9.
17. Frost AE, Farber HW, Barst RJ, et al. Demographics and outcomes of patients diagnosed with pulmonary hypertension with pulmonary capillary wedge pressures 16 to 18 mm Hg: insights from the REVEAL Registry. Chest. 2013;143:185–95.
18. Robbins IM, Hemnes AR, Pugh ME, et al. High prevalence of occult pulmonary venous hypertension revealed by fluid challenge in pulmonary hypertension. Circ Heart Fail. 2014;7: 116–22.
19. Vachiéry J, Adir Y, Barberà JA, et al. Pulmonary hypertension due to left heart diseases. J Am Coll Cardiol. 2013;62:D100–8.
20. Seeger W, Adir Y, Barberà JA, et al. Pulmonary hypertension in chronic lung diseases. J Am Coll Cardiol. 2013;62:D109–16.
21. Wilkens H, Lang I, Blankenburg T, et al. Chronic thromboembolic pulmonary hypertension – a position paper. Dtsch Med Wochenschr. 2014;139:2204–6.
22. Kim NH, Delcroix M, Jenkins DP, et al. Chronic thromboembolic pulmonary hypertension. J Am Coll Cardiol. 2013;62:D92–9.
23. Naeije R, Vachiery J, Yerly P, et al. The transpulmonary pressure gradient for the diagnosis of pulmonary vascular disease. Eur Respir J. 2013;41:217–23.
24. Gerges C, Gerges M, Lang MB, et al. Diastolic pulmonary vascular pressure gradient: a predictor of prognosis in "out-of-proportion" pulmonary hypertension. Chest. 2013;143:758–66.
25. Ghio S, Gavazzi A, Campana C, et al. Independent and additive prognostic value of right ventricular systolic function and pulmonary artery pressure in patients with chronic heart failure. J Am Coll Cardiol. 2001;37:183–8.

26. Oudiz RJ. Pulmonary hypertension associated with left-sided heart disease. Clin Chest Med. 2007;28:233–41.
27. Andersen KH, Iversen M, Kjaergaard J, et al. Prevalence, predictors, and survival in pulmonary hypertension related to end-stage chronic obstructive pulmonary disease. J Heart Lung Transplant. 2012;31:373–80.
28. Shorr AF, Wainright JL, Cors CS, et al. Pulmonary hypertension in patients with pulmonary fibrosis awaiting lung transplant. Eur Respir J. 2007;30:715–21.
29. Cottin V, Le Pavec J, Prévot G, et al. Pulmonary hypertension in patients with combined pulmonary fibrosis and emphysema syndrome. Eur Respir J. 2010;35:105–11.
30. Chaouat A, Bugnet A, Kadaoui N, et al. Severe pulmonary hypertension and chronic obstructive pulmonary disease. Am J Respir Crit Care Med. 2005;172:189–94.
31. Hoeper MM, Andreas S, Bastian A, et al. Pulmonary hypertension due to chronic lung disease: updated Recommendations of the Cologne Consensus Conference 2011. Int J Cardiol. 2011;154 Suppl 1:S45–53.
32. Lange TJ, Baron M, Seiler I, et al. Outcome of patients with severe PH due to lung disease with and without targeted therapy. Cardiovasc Ther. 2014;32:202–8.
33. Lettieri CJ, Nathan SD, Barnett SD, et al. Prevalence and outcomes of pulmonary arterial hypertension in advanced idiopathic pulmonary fibrosis. Chest. 2006;129:746–52.
34. Rycroft CE, Heyes A, Lanza L, et al. Epidemiology of chronic obstructive pulmonary disease: a literature review. Int J Chron Obstruct Pulmon Dis. 2012;7:457–94.
35. Raghu G, Weycker D, Edelsberg J, et al. Incidence and prevalence of idiopathic pulmonary fibrosis. Am J Respir Crit Care Med. 2006;174:810–6.
36. Nathan SD, Shlobin OA, Ahmad S, et al. Serial development of pulmonary hypertension in patients with idiopathic pulmonary fibrosis. Respiration. 2008;76:288–94.
37. Pepke-Zaba J, Delcroix M, Lang I, et al. Chronic thromboembolic pulmonary hypertension (CTEPH): results from an international prospective registry. Circulation. 2011;124:1973–81.
38. Taboada D, Pepke-Zaba J, Jenkins DP, et al. Outcome of pulmonary endarterectomy in symptomatic chronic thromboembolic disease. Eur Respir J. 2014;44:1635–45.
39. Klok FA, van Kralingen KW, van Dijk APJ, et al. Prospective cardiopulmonary screening program to detect chronic thromboembolic pulmonary hypertension in patients after acute pulmonary embolism. Haematologica. 2010;95:970–5.
40. Pengo V, Lensing AWA, Prins MH, et al. Incidence of chronic thromboembolic pulmonary hypertension after pulmonary embolism. N Engl J Med. 2004;350:2257–64.
41. Lewczuk J, Piszko P, Jagas J, et al. Prognostic factors in medically treated patients with chronic pulmonary embolism. Chest. 2001;119:818–23.
42. Jamieson SW, Kapelanski DP, Sakakibara N, et al. Pulmonary endarterectomy: experience and lessons learned in 1,500 cases. Ann Thorac Surg. 2003;76:1457–62.
43. Mayer E, Jenkins D, Lindner J, et al. Surgical management and outcome of patients with chronic thromboembolic pulmonary hypertension: results from an international prospective registry. J Thorac Cardiovasc Surg. 2011;141:702–10.
44. Condliffe R, Kiely DG, Gibbs JSR, et al. Improved outcomes in medically and surgically treated chronic thromboembolic pulmonary hypertension. Am J Respir Crit Care Med. 2008;177:1122–7.
45. Brown LM, Chen H, Halpern S, et al. Delay in recognition of pulmonary arterial hypertension: factors identified from the REVEAL Registry. Chest. 2011;140:19–26.
46. Fisher MR, Forfia PR, Chamera E, et al. Accuracy of Doppler echocardiography in the hemodynamic assessment of pulmonary hypertension. Am J Respir Crit Care Med. 2009;179:615–21.
47. Rich JD, Shah SJ, Swamy RS, et al. Inaccuracy of Doppler echocardiographic estimates of pulmonary artery pressures in patients with pulmonary hypertension: implications for clinical practice. Chest. 2011;139:988–93.
48. Lange TJ, Baumgartner S, Arzt M, et al. Qualitative echocardiography parameters for prediction of pulmonary hypertension. Int J Clin Pract Suppl. 2013;179:5–12.
49. Dornia C, Lange TJ, Behrens G, et al. Multidetector computed tomography for detection and characterization of pulmonary hypertension in consideration of WHO classification. J Comput Assist Tomogr. 2012;36:175–80.

50. Truong QA, Massaro JM, Rogers IS, et al. Reference values for normal pulmonary artery dimensions by noncontrast cardiac computed tomography: the Framingham Heart Study. Circ Cardiovasc Imaging. 2012;5:147–54.
51. King MA, Ysrael M, Bergin CJ. Chronic thromboembolic pulmonary hypertension: CT findings. AJR Am J Roentgenol. 1998;170:955–60.
52. Tunariu N, Gibbs SJR, Win Z, et al. Ventilation-perfusion scintigraphy is more sensitive than multidetector CTPA in detecting chronic thromboembolic pulmonary disease as a treatable cause of pulmonary hypertension. J Nucl Med. 2007;48:680–4.
53. Le Duc-Pennec A, Le Roux P, Cornily J, et al. Diagnostic accuracy of single-photon emission tomography ventilation/perfusion lung scan in the diagnosis of pulmonary embolism. Chest. 2012;141:381–7.
54. Hartmann IJ, Hagen PJ, Melissant CF, et al. Diagnosing acute pulmonary embolism: effect of chronic obstructive pulmonary disease on the performance of D-dimer testing, ventilation/perfusion scintigraphy, spiral computed tomographic angiography, and conventional angiography. ANTELOPE Study Group. Advances in New Technologies Evaluating the Localization of Pulmonary Embolism. Am J Respir Crit Care Med. 2000;162:2232–7.
55. Nakazawa T, Watanabe Y, Hori Y, et al. Lung perfused blood volume images with dual-energy computed tomography for chronic thromboembolic pulmonary hypertension: correlation to scintigraphy with single-photon emission computed tomography. J Comput Assist Tomogr. 2011;35:590–5.
56. McLure LER, Peacock AJ. Cardiac magnetic resonance imaging for the assessment of the heart and pulmonary circulation in pulmonary hypertension. Eur Respir J. 2009;33:1454–66.
57. Kovacs G, Avian A, Olschewski A, et al. Zero reference level for right heart catheterisation. Eur Respir J. 2013;42:1586–94.
58. Montani D, Savale L, Natali D, et al. Long-term response to calcium-channel blockers in non-idiopathic pulmonary arterial hypertension. Eur Heart J. 2010;31:1898–907.
59. Lam CSP, Borlaug BA, Kane GC, et al. Age-associated increases in pulmonary artery systolic pressure in the general population. Circulation. 2009;119:2663–70.
60. Pugh ME, Sivarajan L, Wang L, et al. Causes of pulmonary hypertension in the elderly. Chest. 2014;146:159–66.
61. Galiè N, Corris PA, Frost A, et al. Updated treatment algorithm of pulmonary arterial hypertension. J Am Coll Cardiol. 2013;62:D60–72.
62. Mereles D, Ehlken N, Kreuscher S, et al. Exercise and respiratory training improve exercise capacity and quality of life in patients with severe chronic pulmonary hypertension. Circulation. 2006;114:1482–9.
63. Ivy DD, Abman SH, Barst RJ, et al. Pediatric pulmonary hypertension. J Am Coll Cardiol. 2013;62:D117–26.
64. Olsson KM, Delcroix M, Ghofrani HA, et al. Anticoagulation and survival in pulmonary arterial hypertension: results from the Comparative, Prospective Registry of Newly Initiated Therapies for Pulmonary Hypertension (COMPERA). Circulation. 2014;129:57–65.
65. Sitbon O, Humbert M, Jaïs X, et al. Long-term response to calcium channel blockers in idiopathic pulmonary arterial hypertension. Circulation. 2005;111:3105–11.
66. Rich S, Kaufmann E, Levy PS. The effect of high doses of calcium-channel blockers on survival in primary pulmonary hypertension. N Engl J Med. 1992;327:76–81.
67. Sitbon O, Humbert M, Jagot JL, et al. Inhaled nitric oxide as a screening agent for safely identifying responders to oral calcium-channel blockers in primary pulmonary hypertension. Eur Respir J. 1998;12:265–70.
68. Hoeper MM, Markevych I, Spiekerkoetter E, et al. Goal-oriented treatment and combination therapy for pulmonary arterial hypertension. Eur Respir J. 2005;26:858–63.
69. Pulido T, Adzerikho I, Channick RN, et al. Macitentan and morbidity and mortality in pulmonary arterial hypertension. N Engl J Med. 2013;369:809–18.
70. Ghofrani H, Galiè N, Grimminger F, et al. Riociguat for the treatment of pulmonary arterial hypertension. N Engl J Med. 2013;369:330–40.

71. McLaughlin VV, Gaine SP, Howard LS, et al. Treatment goals of pulmonary hypertension. J Am Coll Cardiol. 2013;62:D73–81.
72. Wensel R, Francis DP, Meyer FJ, et al. Incremental prognostic value of cardiopulmonary exercise testing and resting haemodynamics in pulmonary arterial hypertension. Int J Cardiol. 2013;167:1193–8.
73. Lange TJ, Keller A, Arzt M, et al. Six-minute walk distance target in elderly patients with idiopathic pulmonary arterial hypertension – consideration of predicted values. Int J Clin Pract. 2014;68:543–50.
74. Califf RM, Adams KF, McKenna WJ, et al. A randomized controlled trial of epoprostenol therapy for severe congestive heart failure: The Flolan International Randomized Survival Trial (FIRST). Am Heart J. 1997;134:44–54.
75. Guazzi M, Vicenzi M, Arena R, et al. PDE5 inhibition with sildenafil improves left ventricular diastolic function, cardiac geometry, and clinical status in patients with stable systolic heart failure: results of a 1-year, prospective, randomized, placebo-controlled study. Circ Heart Fail. 2011;4:8–17.
76. Redfield MM, Chen HH, Borlaug BA, et al. Effect of phosphodiesterase-5 inhibition on exercise capacity and clinical status in heart failure with preserved ejection fraction: a randomized clinical trial. JAMA. 2013;309:1268–77.
77. Held M, Walthelm J, Baron S, et al. Functional impact of pulmonary hypertension due to hypoventilation and changes under noninvasive ventilation. Eur Respir J. 2014;43:156–65.
78. Zieliński J, Tobiasz M, Hawryłkiewicz I, et al. Effects of long-term oxygen therapy on pulmonary hemodynamics in COPD patients: a 6-year prospective study. Chest. 1998;113:65–70.
79. Oswald-Mammosser M, Weitzenblum E, Quoix E, et al. Prognostic factors in COPD patients receiving long-term oxygen therapy. Importance of pulmonary artery pressure. Chest. 1995; 107:1193–8.
80. Ghofrani HA, Wiedemann R, Rose F, et al. Sildenafil for treatment of lung fibrosis and pulmonary hypertension: a randomised controlled trial. Lancet. 2002;360:895–900.
81. Collard HR, Anstrom KJ, Schwarz MI, et al. Sildenafil improves walk distance in idiopathic pulmonary fibrosis. Chest. 2007;131:897–9.
82. Zisman DA, Schwarz M, Anstrom KJ, et al. A controlled trial of sildenafil in advanced idiopathic pulmonary fibrosis. N Engl J Med. 2010;363:620–8.
83. Olschewski H, Ghofrani HA, Walmrath D, et al. Inhaled prostacyclin and iloprost in severe pulmonary hypertension secondary to lung fibrosis. Am J Respir Crit Care Med. 1999;160: 600–7.
84. Piazza G, Goldhaber SZ. Chronic thromboembolic pulmonary hypertension. N Engl J Med. 2011;364:351–60.
85. Ghofrani H, D'Armini AM, Grimminger F, et al. Riociguat for the treatment of chronic thromboembolic pulmonary hypertension. N Engl J Med. 2013;369:319–29.
86. Feinstein JA, Goldhaber SZ, Lock JE, et al. Balloon pulmonary angioplasty for treatment of chronic thromboembolic pulmonary hypertension. Circulation. 2001;103:10–3.
87. Mizoguchi H, Ogawa A, Munemasa M, et al. Refined balloon pulmonary angioplasty for inoperable patients with chronic thromboembolic pulmonary hypertension. Circ Cardiovasc Interv. 2012;5:748–55.

Chapter 10
Antiplatelet Therapy in Elderly Patients

Andreas May

Dual antiplatelet therapy (DAPT) using aspirin and an oral P2Y12 receptor (ADP receptor) blocker is the current standard regimen to prevent atherothrombotic events in patients after percutaneous coronary stenting [1]. However, there is an ongoing debate on the best antithrombotic therapy after coronary interventions regarding the best choice of antiplatelet drug combination, dosage, and duration [2]. The decision needs to take multiple factors into account including the individual patient risk for ischemic events (e.g., stent thrombosis) as well as for bleeding. Albeit the numerical incidence is low, the consequences of stent thrombosis are severe with a 64 % rate of death and myocardial infarction and a mortality rate of 9–45 % [3, 4].

The risk for ischemic events appears to depend on the clinical setting (stable, ACS-NSTE, STEMI), the urgency and mode of the intervention, the respective stent type, comorbidities and the procedural result. The risk for bleeding depends on a potential need for anticoagulation and on individual patient characteristics (e.g., age), which can be quantified by the so-called HASBLED score (Table 10.1) [5].

Current standard guidelines recommend DAPT for a time span from 4 weeks in patients undergoing elective stenting using bare metal stents (BMS) up to 12 months in patients with drug eluting stents (DES) and/or patients undergoing coronary stenting for acute coronary syndrome [1]. These recommendations do not adequately apply to patients with enhanced bleeding risk or patients with indication for additional oral anticoagulation in whom the recommended duration of DAPT ranges from 2–4 weeks to 12 months depending on the individual risk profile [4, 7]. Specific procedural aspects (suboptimal result, bifurcational stenting) that may hinder a complete endothelialization of the stent may even legitimate a prolonged DAPT

A. May
Department of Internal Medicine, Klinikum Memmingen,
Memmingen, Germany
e-mail: andreas.may@klinikum-memmingen.de

H. Rittger (ed.), *Interventional Cardiology in the Elderly*,
DOI 10.1007/978-3-319-21142-8_10

Table 10.1 HASBLED score for calculation of the individual patient risk for bleeding and CHA_2DS_2VASc-score for calculation of the risk for thromboembolism in patients with atrial fibrillation [5, 6]

Letter	Clinical characteristic	Points
H	Hypertension	1
A	Abnormal renal and liver enzymes (1 point each)	1–2
S	Stroke	1
B	Bleeding	1
L	Labile INRs	1
E	*Elderly (e.g. age >65 years)*	*1*
D	Drugs or alcohol (1 point each)	1–2
Maximum score		9

Letter	Clinical characteristic	Points
C	Congestive heart failure/left ventricular dysfunction	1
H	Hypertension	1
A_2	*Age ≥ 75 years*	*2*
D	Diabetes	1
S_2	Stroke/TIA/thromboembolism	2
V	Vascular disease (prior myocardial Infarction; peripheral artery disease)	1
A	*Age 65–74 years*	*1*
Sc	Sex category (female)	1
Maximum score		9

>1 year in individual patients [7]. The emerging diversity of next generation stent platforms (e.g., bioabsorbable scaffolds) further contributes to the need of a more and more individualized decision process.

Age plays an essential role for the final decision of how to treat the individual patient after PCI. Elderly patients carry an increased risk of bleeding when taking anticoagulation or antiplatelet therapy or even a combination of both (Table 10.1). Factors that may account for the enhanced bleeding risk are the higher incidence of comorbidities, frailty, low body weight, and the increased need for unplanned non-cardiac surgery.

The choice of the antithrombotic therapy in elderly patients remains an ongoing challenge, because they – besides enhanced risk for bleeding – often require an even more intensified antithrombotic therapy as compared to younger patients: First, elderly patients more often present with acute coronary syndromes requiring prolonged dual antiplatelet therapy. Second, the incidence of atrial fibrillation increases with age as does the risk of stroke in patients with atrial fibrillation [6], which can be calculated by the CHA_2DS_2Vasc Score (Table 10.1). Therefore, despite having an increased risk of bleeding, elderly patients undergoing coronary stent implantation often require an effective anticoagulation in combination with antiplatelet therapy [5, 7, 8].

Patients with Stable Coronary Artery Disease Without Recent PCI

Patients with symptomatic, stable coronary artery disease (CAD) are – irrespective of any prior PCI – advised to take antiplatelet monotherapy. This recommendation is based on data from multiple large trials performed in the 1980s and 1990s, e.g., a metaanalysis of the so-called antithrombotic trialist's collaboration. This trial proved the superiority of antiplatelet therapy versus placebo in patients with symptomatic coronary artery disease regarding the incidence of stroke, myocardial infarction or death [9]. The CAPRIE Trial has additionally compared the treatment of aspirin (325 mg/day) with clopidogrel (75 mg/day) in 19,185 patients with symptomatic atherothrombotic disease history of stroke, myocardial infarction or symptomatic peripheral artery disease [10]. This trial showed the non-inferiority of clopidogrel, which may serve as an alternative to aspirin in these patients. In fact, CAPRIE even showed a benefit for clopidogrel in the subgroup of patients with peripheral arterial disease regarding the incidence of ischemic stroke, myocardial infarction or vascular death. However, dual antiplatelet therapy (DAPT) did not show a clinical benefit over antiplatelet monotherapy in clinically stable patients: CHARISMA studied the potential benefit of a combined dual antiplatelet therapy using low-dose aspirin (75 mg/day) plus clopdogrel (75 mg/day) versus aspirin monotherapy in 15,603 patients with symptomatic cardiovascular disease or with multiple risk factors and followed them over a period of 28 months (median). CHARISMA did not show any additional benefit for dual antiplatelet therapy regarding the incidence of ischemic events, however, a trend of enhanced bleeding events with dual therapy [11].

Together, the current recommendation for patients with symptomatic stable coronary disease (without recent PCI) is a lifelong antiplatelet monotherapy using aspirin (75–125 mg/day) or – as an alternative – clopidogrel (75 mg/day) irrespective of any additional risk factors [1].

Patients with Coronary Stent Implantation in Stable Angina

Stent thrombosis is the most severe complication, and, therefore, is the Achilles'heel of coronary stent implantation. In patients with coronary stent implantation, dual antiplatelet therapy using acetylsalicylic acid (ASA, aspirin) and an ADP receptor antagonist (e.g., clopidogrel) is the current standard strategy to prevent stent thrombosis.

DAPT Initiation and "Loading dose"

Since clopidogrel is a "pro-drug", which requires metabolization in the liver, clopidogrel should be administered prior to the intervention. Depending on the time interval from the intake of the "loading dose" to the planned coronary intervention, it is currently recommended to use a loading dose of at least 300 (>12 h prior to PCI) or 600 mg (<3 h) prior to a planned PCI [1]. The best time point of administration of clopidogrel is currently a matter of debate. In patients undergoing coronary angiography for stable angina it is recommended to start clopidogrel "loading" after the diagnostic angiography on the table immediately prior to PCI. Besides clopidogrel dual antiplatelet therapy also includes a 150–300 mg oral loading dose of ASA (or 80–150 mg i.v.).

DAPT Dosage and Duration

ASA is recommended to be taken life-long by 75–100 mg per os daily, the recommended dosage of clopidogrel is 75 mg daily [12–14].

The recommended duration of DAPT is a matter of an ongoing debate. It depends on several conditions, e.g., stent type (bare metal or drug-eluting stent), the individual angiographic result, clinical condition (elective stenting versus stenting in ACS), as well as additional individual patient characteristics (e.g., age, history of bleeding).

DAPT is recommended for at least 1 month after BMS implantation and for 6 months after DES implantation by the European Society of Cardiology [1]. Having the second and third generation DES available the risk of stent thrombosis has been further reduced in the meantime. Recently, it has been shown that a period of 3 months of DAPT may be sufficient in selected patients with selected next generation DES [15, 16].

Nevertheless, the development and clinical application of novel stent or "scaffold" designs using novel bioresorbable materials requires additional clinical experience and investigations.

Accordingly, the ESC recommends to make the decision on the respective duration of DAPT after DES implantation on an individual basis: One may consider a shorter DAPT duration (<6 months) after DES implantation in patients at high bleeding risk and a longer duration (>6 months) in patients at high ischaemic and low bleeding risk (class IIb recommendation) [1]. In elderly patients these considerations need to be taken into account.

Patients with Coronary Stent Implantation in Acute Coronary Syndromes

Patients with acute coronary syndromes have an increased immediate risk for ischemic complications as well thereafter. Therefore, these patients generally require an intensified dual antiplatelet therapy from the time of hospitalization and PCI over a period of 12 months [1].

The acute coronary syndrome (ACS) comprises a large clinical spectrum from unstable angina, non-ST elevation myocardial infarction (NSTEMI) to ST-elevation myocardial infarction (STEMI). The ACS is pathophysiologically characterized by a combination of a progredient atherosclerosis with the formation of plaques and arterial thrombosis caused by plaque rupture. Therefore, an optimised and well balanced antithrombotic therapy plays a crucial role in the therapy of ACS. This is important both in patients treated medically and in patients treated by a PCI.

Antiplatelet therapy plays a key role in the treatment of both the acute and the chronic phase of the ACS. Various pharmacologic options exist to inhibit different activation pathways of platelets:

Acetylsalicylic Acid (ASA)

ASA is the classical drug for platelet inhibition. In patients with unstable angina, data reveal that ASA exerts a highly significant cardioprotective effect. Even a short-term treatment reduces the incidence of ischemic events. The maximum protective effect is apparently achieved at a daily dose of merely 75 mg. The current dose recommendations for acute coronary syndrome are 75–150 mg /day [1]. Higher doses do not have an additional protective benefit, however increase the incidence of severe bleeding events [17].

In patients with acute myocardial infarction with or without lysis therapy, the two large international studies ISIS-2 and ISIS-3 provided the most convincing evidence for the preventative efficacy of ASA [18, 19]. The sole administration of ASA reduced the number of deaths by 23 % ($p<0.00001$) in comparison to placebo. In addition, ASA reduced the incidence of non-fatal reinfarction and stroke by 50 %. In contrast to treatment with streptokinase, no increase in cerebral hemorrhage was observed under ASA. Streptokinase alone also reduced the mortality highly significantly by 25 %, but led to an increase in the reinfarction rate of 30 %. This increase was not observed under the combination therapy with ASA. The combination of streptokinase with ASA has a significantly better efficacy than each of the substances given as monotherapy (reduction in mortality by 42 % compared to placebo). This allows the conclusion that the simultaneous inhibition of platelet function makes a central contribution to the success of antithrombotic treatment for myocardial infarction. According to the ISIS-3 study, the additional treatment with heparin in comparison to ASA monotherapy is not able to improve the survival rate but does significantly increase the number of hemorrhagic complications. In summary, the recommended dose in acute therapy is 160–325 mg ASA. For an ongoing therapy, a dose of 75–100 mg ASA has been proven safe and effective.

P2Y12 Receptor Antagonists

In ACS, P2Y12 receptor antagonists, e.g., clopidogrel, prasugrel or ticagrelor, should be combined with ASA yielding a so-called dual antiplatelet therapy (DAPT). The ADP-Receptor antagonists are effective in patients with clinical manifestations of atherosclerosis that involve the coronary, cerebral, or peripheral arterial circulation. They show promise when combined with ASA, probably due to the blockade of complementary activation pathways in platelets.

Clopidogrel

The efficacy of dual antiplatelet therapy in NSTE-ACS has been proved in the CURE study (Clopidogrel in Unstable Angina to Prevent Recurrent Ischemic Events) [20]. Patients with NSTE-ACS received aspirin monotherapy or a combination of aspirin and clopidogrel (initially 300 mg followed by 75 mg/day) over a period of 9–12 months. The patients treated with the dual antiplatelet therapy showed a significant reduction of the combined endpoint (cardiovascular death, nonfatal myocardial infarction, stroke; 9.3 vs. 11.3 %). The analysis of the interventionally treated subgroup (PCI-Cure) demonstrated a relative risk reduction of 31 % concerning cardiovascular death or myocardial infarction [21]. A subgroup analysis of CHARISMA [11] additionally showed that patients with AMI benefit from a long-term dual antiplatelet therapy with respect to ischemic events without an enhanced rate of bleeding.

Clinical limitations of clopidogrel use are its delayed begin of effect but also its individually variable magnitude of effect. For acceleration of effect, higher "loading" doses of clopidogrel have been suggested and investigated. In conclusion, a loading dose of 600 mg has demonstrated to be more effective than 300 mg in terms of rapid and stronger efficacy. In patients with ACS clopidogrel is currently only recommended, when the novel and stronger substances prasugrel and ticagrelor are not indicated or not available (Class I, level B recommendation) [1]. In those patients, a daily dose of 75 mg of clopidogrel is recommended for the duration of 12 months irrespective of the initial way of treatment unless there are contraindications such as excessive risk of bleeding.

Prasugrel

Prasugrel (60 mg loading and 10 mg daily maintenance dose) is a prodrug that irreversibly blocks the P2Y12 receptor with a faster onset and a stronger and a more reliable antiplatelet inhibition as compared to clopidogrel. The clinical efficacy of prasugrel in acute coronary syndromes was proved in the TRITON TIMI 38 trial against the 300 mg loading dose of clopidogrel—both started in the catheterization laboratory after diagnostic angiography [8]. Prasugrel proved beneficial regarding a composite ischaemic outcome: Cardiovascular events were reduced in prasugrel-treated patients (9.3 % versus 11.2 %; $P<0.002$), which was mainly driven by a significantly decreased incidence of myocardial infarction (7.1 % vs. 9.2 %; $p>0.001$). However, severe bleeding complications were enhanced with prasugrel compared to clopidogrel (TIMI non-CABG major bleeding 1.8 % vs. 2.4 %, $p<0.03$).

Notably, patients at high risk for ischemic events such as patients with STEMI or with NSTEMI and diabetes showed profound benefit from prasugrel without significantly affecting major bleeding. On the other hand, patients with a history of transient ischemic attack or stroke, body weight <60 kg or elderly patients (≥75 years) showed enhanced bleeding events and, accordingly, should not be treated with prasugrel. Consequently, patients with acute coronary syndromes, known coronary angiography, and planned PCI are recommended to take prasugrel for 12 months with a Class I / Level B [1].

Prasugrel is generally not recommended for patients of ≥75 years of age in its standard dose. If, after a careful individual risk–benefit evaluation, therapy is judged necessary in the ≥75 years age or low body weight (60 kg) groups then, following a loading dose of 60 mg, a reduced maintenance dose of 5 mg may be prescribed.

Ticagrelor

Alternatively, ticagrelor can be administered in patients with ACS using 180 mg loading dose followed by 90 mg twice daily. Ticagrelor is a cyclopentyltriazolopyrimidine, is an oral and reversibly binding P2Y12 receptor blocker with a plasma half-life of approximately 6–12 h. The Study of Platelet Inhibition and Patient Outcomes (PLATO) study randomly assigned ACS patients—with or without prior loading with clopidogrel and irrespective of the strategy (invasive vs. non-invasive) – to treatment with ticagrelor or clopidogrel [22]. The study demonstrated significantly superior results for ticagrelor in the composite ischaemic endpoint (9.8 % vs. 11.7 %; p<0.001) and mortality (4.0 % vs. 5.1 %; p<0.001). Major bleeding occurred in 5.3 % of the patients in the ticagrelor group and in 5.8 % in the clopidogrel group. There was no difference in the overall rates of fatal haemorrhage (0.3 % in both groups) despite a higher rate of fatal intracranial haemorrhage in the ticagrelor group (0.1 % vs. 0.001 %; P<0.02). Ticagrelor was associated with an increased rate of adverse effects including dyspnoea, increased frequency of ventricular pauses, and asymptomatic increases in uric acid.

A substudy of PLATO has investigated the subgroup of elderly patients in PLATO [23]. The significant clinical benefit and overall safety of ticagrelor compared with clopidogrel in ACS patients in the PLATO cohort were not found to depend on age.

Conclusion

The current international guidelines of the European Society of Cardiology (ESC) recommend all patients with ACS to initially get ASA at an oral loading dose of 150–300 mg (or 80–150 mg i.v.) and a maintenance dose of 75–100 mg daily long-term regardless of the treatment strategy (IA) [1]. In addition to ASA, a P2Y12 receptor antagonist should be started and maintained over a period of 12 months unless there are contraindications such as excessive bleeding. Options are:

1. Prasugrel (loading dose 60 mg, daily dose 10 mg) in patients in whom coronary artery is known and who are planned to undergo PCI (if no contraindication exists). In elderly patients (≥75 years) the routine dose is contraindicated, but a reduced daily dose of 5 mg is an option.
2. Ticagrelor (loading dose 180 mg, daily dose 2×90 mg), if no contraindication exists. Ticagrelor is not contraindicated in elderly patients.
3. Clopidogrel (loading dose 600 mg, daily dose 75 mg) only when ticagrelor or prasugrel are not available or contraindicated.

References

1. Kolh P, Windecker S. ESC/EACTS myocardial revascularization guidelines 2014. Eur Heart J. 2014;35(46):3235–6.
2. May AE. Antiplatelet therapy after coronary stenting: for how long? Lancet. 2013; 382(9906):1684–5.
3. Iakovou I, Schmidt T, Bonizzoni E, et al. Incidence, predictors, and outcome of thrombosis after successful implantation of drug-eluting stents. JAMA. 2005;293:2126–30.
4. Grines CL, Bonow RO, Casey DE, et al. Prevention of premature discontinuation of dual antiplatelet therapy in patients with coronary artery stents: a science advisory from the American Heart Association, American College of Cardiology, Society for Cardiovascular Angiography and Interventions, American College of Surgeons, and American Dental Association, with representation from the American College of Physicians. J Am Coll Cardiol. 2007;49:734–9.
5. Pisters R, Lane DA, Nieuwlaat R, de Vos CB, Crijns HJ, Lip GY. A novel user-friendly score (HASBLED) to assess 1-year risk of major bleeding in patients with atrial fibrillation: the Euro Heart Survey. Chest. 2010;138(5):1093–100.
6. Camm AJ, Kirchhof P, Lip GY, et al. Guidelines for the management of atrial fibrillation: the Task Force for the Management of Atrial Fibrillation of the European Society of Cardiology (ESC). Eur Heart J. 2010;31:2369–429.
7. May AE, Geisler T, Gawaz M. Individualized antithrombotic therapy in high risk patients after coronary stenting. A double-edged sword between thrombosis and bleeding. Thromb Haemost. 2008;99:487–93.
8. Wiviott SD, Braunwald E, McCabe CH, TRITONTIMI 38 Investigator. Prasugrel versus clopidogrel in patients with acute coronary syndromes. N Engl J Med. 2007;357:2001–15.
9. Antithrombotic Trialists' Collaboration. Collaborative meta-analysis of randomised trials of antiplatelet therapy for prevention of death, myocardial infarction, and stroke in high risk patients. BMJ. 2002;324:71–83.
10. CAPRIE Steering Committee. A randomised, blinded, trial of clopidogrel versus aspirin in patients at risk of ischaemic events (CAPRIE). Lancet. 1996;348(9038):1329–39.
11. Bhatt DL, Fox KA, Hacke W, Berger PB, Black HR, Boden WE, Cacoub P, Cohen EA, Creager MA, Easton JD, Flather MD, Haffner SM, Hamm CW, Hankey GJ, Johnston SC, Mak KH, Mas JL, Montalescot G, Pearson TA, Steg PG, Steinhubl SR, Weber MA, Brennan DM, Fabry-Ribaudo L, Booth J, Topol EJ, CHARISMA Investigators. Clopidogrel and aspirin versus aspirin alone for the prevention of atherothrombotic events. N Engl J Med. 2006;354(16):1706–17.
12. Silber S, Albertsson P, Aviles FF, Camici PG, Colombo A, Hamm C, Jorgensen E, Marco J, Nordrehaug JE, Ruzyllo W, Urban P, Stone GW, Wijns W. Guidelines for percutaneous coronary interventions. The task force for percutaneous coronary interventions of the European Society of Cardiology. Eur Heart J. 2005;26:804–47.
13. Patrono C, Andreotti F, Arnesen H, Badimon L, Baigent C, Collet JP, De Caterina R, Gulba D, Huber K, Husted S, Kristensen SD, Morais J, Neumann FJ, Rasmussen LH, Siegbahn A, Steg

PG, Storey RF, Van deWerf F, Verheugt F. Antiplatelet agents for the treatment and prevention of atherothrombosis. Eur Heart J. 2011;32(23):2922–32.

14. Patrono C, Rodriguez LA, Landolfi R, Baigent C. Low-dose aspirin for the prevention of atherothrombosis. N Engl J Med. 2005;353:2373–83.
15. Feres F, Costa RA, Abizaid A, Leon MB, Marin-Neto JA, Botelho RV, King SB, Negoita M, Liu M, de Paula JE, Mangione JA, Meireles GX, Castello HJ, Nicolela E, Perin MA, Devito FS, Labrunie A, Salvadori D, Gusmão M, Staico R, Costa JR, de Castro JP, Abizaid AS, Bhatt DL. Three vs.twelve months of dual antiplatelet therapy after zotarolimus-eluting stents: the OPTIMIZE Randomized Trial. JAMA. 2013;310(23):2510–22.
16. Kim BK, Hong MK, Shin DH, Nam CM, Kim JS, Ko YG, Choi D, Kang TS, Park BE, Kang WC, Lee SH, Yoon JH, Hong BK, Kwon HM, Jang Y. A new strategy for discontinuation of dual antiplatelet therapy: the RESET Trial (REal Safety and Efficacy of 3-month dual antiplatelet Therapy following Endeavor zotarolimus-eluting stent implantation). J Am Coll Cardiol. 2012;60(15):1340–8.
17. Berger JS. Aspirin, clopidogrel, and ticagrelor in acute coronary syndromes. Am J Cardiol. 2013;112(5):737–45.
18. ISIS-2 (Second International Study of Infarct Survival) Collaborative Group. Randomized trial of intravenous streptokinase, oral aspirin, both, or neither among 17,187 cases of suspected acute myocardial infarction: ISIS-2. J Am Coll Cardiol. 1988;12:3A–13.
19. ISIS-3: A randomised comparison of streptokinase vs tissue plasminogen activator vs anistreplase and of aspirin plus heparin vs aspirin alone among 41,299 cases of suspected acute myocardial infarction. ISIS-3 (Third International Study of Infarct Survival) Collaborative Group. Lancet 1992;339(8796):753–70.
20. Mehta SR. Aspirin and clopidogrel in patients with ACS undergoing PCI: CURE and PCI-CURE. J Invasive Cardiol. 2003;15(Suppl B):17B–20.
21. Mehta SR, Yusuf S, Peters RJ, et al., Clopidogrel in Unstable angina to prevent Recurrent Events trial (CURE) Investigators. Effects of pre-treatment with clopidogrel and aspirin followed by long-term therapy in patients undergoing percutaneous coronary intervention: the PCI-CURE study. Lancet. 2001;358:527–33.
22. Wallentin L, Becker RC, Budaj A, et al., for the PLATO Investigators. Ticagrelor versus clopidogrel in patients with acute coronary syndromes. N Engl J Med. 2009;361:1045–57.
23. Husted S, James S, Becker RC, Horrow J, Katus H, Storey RF, Cannon CP, Heras M, Lopes RD, Morais J, Mahaffey KW, Bach RG, Wojdyla D, Wallentin L, PLATO Study Group. Ticagrelor versus clopidogrel in elderly patients with acute coronary syndromes: a substudy from the prospective randomized PLATelet inhibition and patient Outcomes (PLATO) trial. Circ Cardiovasc Qual Outcomes. 2012;5(5):680–8.

Chapter 11
Ethical Aspects of Interventional Cardiology in Geriatric Patients

Thomas Frühwald

In the past years medicine has achieved amazing progress in diagnostic and therapeutic interventions, particularly in new technologies expanding the boundaries of the possible, of the "doable", nurturing hopes and expectations of alleviating burdensome symptoms, of curing conditions that in the not so far past were considered to have a grim prognosis.

Many of these conditions are associated with advanced age. Geriatric patients are becoming a prime target group for new interventions promising them more years of life enjoyed in good quality, acceptable condition and function, self determined and autonomous. Deciding about medical diagnostic and therapeutic interventions for and with geriatric patients may present some particular ethical challenges.

Ethics is a fundamental part of geriatric medicine. Ethical questions are important in all fields of medicine, but in geriatrics they are of particular importance. This branch of medicine is concerned with the care of health problems of mostly very old people close to the end of their life. They are physically, mentally and socially vulnerable – frail – individuals with a high risk for progressive deficits in physical and cognitive functions, thus progressively dependent on help and care.

Decisions about medical interventions are easier when the patients concerned have an intact decisional capacity. This situation becomes more complex and difficult when dealing with multimorbid, frequently cognitively impaired very old individuals.

Ethics is about systematically asking the right questions [15]. *This process should be logically structured, questions may remain unanswered. It is about questioning prejudices and modes of action, it means explaining terminology, requesting the best facts possible, formulating definitions, and helping to reflect a problem. Good ethics begins with good facts, with good evidence – not with groundless assumptions.*

T. Frühwald
Geriatric Acute Care Department, Krankenhaus Hietzing mit Neurologischem Zentrum Rosenhügel, Wien, Austria
e-mail: thomas.fruehwald@wienkav.at

H. Rittger (ed.), *Interventional Cardiology in the Elderly*,
DOI 10.1007/978-3-319-21142-8_11

An ethical problem consists basically of the question of what should be done, not what can be done. In this context fits a citation by Jean-Pierre Junod, a pioneer of European geriatrics:

> The desire to dominate the medical situation by all means is only the expression of a misguided striving for success. Our medical knowledge is often beyond the real expectations of the aged patient. In geriatrics the physician, the nurse, the therapist frequently have to accept being guided by the patient. Dominating the aged patient physically and emotionally, disregarding his or her dignity, neglecting his or her general needs are at the origin of many ills. Failing to share the same hopes and aspirations may result in the danger of being able to dominate only one's own ambitions. [11]

The seemingly most important questions concern situations in which life or death decisions have to be made: should one start cardio-pulmonary resuscitation? Should invasive diagnostic and therapeutic interventions be pursued? Should one intubate, should artificial nutrition, should dialysis be started? These question always concern an individual, they are of utmost importance in his or her real life context. The everyday situations with questions arising are apparently less dramatic: Can a patient be discharged home? Should one propose nursing home care? Should a particular, perhaps burdensome therapy be initiated? Is informed consent possible? These questions are best discussed in a multidisciplinary team.

Ethics – Attempts of a Definition

Ethics is a discipline of philosophy. Generally speaking it deals with questions concerning the good and the attitude that should determine human action. Ethics is about questions arising from the interaction between individuals of a society. Using philosophical methods ethics attempts to demonstrate the fundamental principles for a just and meaningful action in living together with others. Ethics is effective when it is about acting with or deciding for other individuals. Ethical principles and justifications should not rely on external authority or convention, they should be applicable universally with reason and sense, and they should take a higher-ranking position than morals [13].

In simpler, more pragmatic terms the Austro-American Physician and Bioethicist Erich H. Loewy explains ethics as a discipline that proposes the question "How should I act when also someone else could be affected?" Ethics theoretically inquires about the "good" and the "bad", but in practice – in most of the situations – it is about he "bad", the "worse" and the "even worse". Ethics is not about the exchange of unfounded arguments, it is concerned with general rules and guidelines as well as with problems in individual cases. Ethics calls for tolerance of other opinions in a human framework [15].

The theologian and ethicist Ulrich Körtner defines ethics as the "self-reflexive theory of morals". That means judging the morality of human action according to the categories of "good" and "bad". Contrary to "ethics", the ancient Greek term "ethos" or the Latin "moralis" describes behavioral norms in a society or a group accepted and stabilized by tradition [12].

Ethics is not an individual's personal morality. One's own conception of morality can be derived from religion, culture, tradition, personal experience and conscience but it will not be the same for a person of another tradition, with different experiences. Ethics attempts to find a common denominator for different world-views, religions and cultures and whenever possible to propose a framework in which different individual moral conceptions can be expressed. Ethics tries to reflect critically and objectively what has been established as moral habit in a society and to look for generally acceptable, objective criteria and rules for modes of behavior. Ethics should question prejudices and established procedures, demand exact definitions, it should help to logically reflect problems, to pose questions in a systematic, structured way. In a secular and pluralistic society ethics should be kept free of all religious and ideological premises [23].

Medical ethics is not only about presenting and discussing individual patient cases, it is not just the application of "moral common sense" of physicians. Medical ethics is no special ethics, it means rather ethics in special situations – like for example ethics in geriatrics. It refers to physicians' actions and to patients' attitudes, to situations common in the hospital, the nursing home, the doctor's office. Beyond that it encompasses ethical problems of institutional actions, like for example issues of distributional justice in the healthcare system [24].

Good ethics needs some prerequisites: first of all it needs a good knowledge basis and good facts. In medicine this means that physicians who are not competent enough in their domain, who do not continuously keep themselves informed, who are not up-to-date with the latest developments in their specialty cannot act also ethically correctly. Good ethics begins with good facts, not with groundless assumptions [16]. Good, ethical decisions are not possible without optimal knowledge and competence in diagnosis, prognosis, and treatment alternatives.

Another aspect to keep in mind is the fact that professionally and ethically good medical action – as Erich Loewy said – does not happen "in a vacuum". The framework in which the physician has to act is determined by the institution (the hospital, the healthcare system) and thus by the society. It is very difficult to act in an ethical way in an institution that is not based on ethical principles. It is equally difficult to build a just, ethical healthcare system in an unjust society [18].

The Importance of Ethical Considerations in Geriatric Medicine

Why should ethical considerations have such a high level of significance particularly in geriatrics? Especially when – as mentioned above – ethics is about the search for basic principles for just, meaningful, judicious, reasonable – in one word: good – action. There are a few explanations:

- Geriatric medicine deals with old, very old, patients who frequently are in need of help and care because of their higher risk for losses of physical, cognitive, emotional and social function. The situation of these vulnerable, frail patients often is not adequately taken care of by our social and healthcare system.

- Geriatric medicine can also be characterized by the fact that it deals with people at the end of their lives. Death is not the absolute adversary in this field of medicine, not necessarily a symbol of failure. In many respects there is concordance between Palliative Care and Geriatrics.
- In Geriatric Medicine patients are being taken care of not only for a more or less limited period of time, but for the whole of the final period of their lives, often in an environment not of their primary choice, like for example in a nursing home.

Therefore, ethics is a fundamental part of geriatric action. This is particularly true when considering frailty, the risk of dependence on help and care by others.

The discussion of ethical problems in geriatrics circles around two poles: one is autonomy, the right of a person to determine his or her own fate, to exert his or her own will – even though taking into account certain limits set by society. With geriatric patients frequently the question arises whether he or she possesses the competence to comprehend and to judge the situation and if he or she has sufficient independent decisional capacity. The other pole is beneficence, the obligation to do well to others, to help minimize suffering. Oftentimes this borders on paternalism – one acts and decides in conflict with the principle of autonomy (see below).

The infantilization of the older person is wrong and unethical, even in the presence of cognitive impairment (dementia) that may lead to a gradual loss of cognitive capacities. But there are variably long individual progressions of cognitive functional deficits between early and advanced stages of dementia. The presence of this diagnosis does not automatically imply an incapacity to comprehend and to chose and decide independently.

Principles of Biomedical Ethics

Present day biomedical ethics is guided by four key considerations proposed by Beauchamp and Childress as moral principles to help focus everyday decisions in medical practice. They are the basis of an ethical system termed "principlism" that guides medical decision-making in our pluralistic society, they provide a basic analytical framework for reflecting on moral issues within biomedicine [2].

These four guiding principles are:

1. **Beneficence**: this principle implies the general human obligation to do good, to act to the benefit of others, for the physician it means the duty to act in the best interest of the individual patient. It demands to weigh the expected benefit of medical interventions against their potential harm – this judgment always has to be done in the decision making process.
2. **Non-Maleficence**: requires to avoid harm and suffering from other individuals, patients. It means the obligation to respect the individual's right to his or her spiritual and physical integrity.

3. **Autonomy**: requires the respect of the individual's right for self-determination as far as his or her personal existential perspectives and concepts go. This is implicit in the rule of informed consent in decision-making by which the patient should be provided with clear information about the expected benefits and risks of the procedure. This principle also implies the physician's duty to help the patient maintain control over his or her medical treatment.
4. **Justice**: this principle obliges to avoid discrimination by irrelevant criteria, to guarantee fairness of access to resources. It means also that patient selection criteria should be as objective as possible, transparent and reproducible.

Tensions and conflicts between these four principles may arise, frequently they cannot be eliminated, and one has to able to tolerate them in a constructive way [4].

The four guiding principles of bioethics should be applied also in interventional cardiology, for example in deciding whether or not to perform a transcatheter aortic valve replacement in geriatric patients [3]. Weighing expected benefit and potential harm for the individual patient, thus following the principles of **beneficence and non-maleficence**, is crucial. When considering such an intervention, the fundamental question is the extent to which the patient's quality of life will be improved. This key question must be considered and discussed with each individual being assessed – thus honoring his or her **autonomy**.

In this respect "what can be done" and "what should be done" are not equivalent questions. A patient's right do die with dignity must be respected. The principle of autonomy also makes **informed consent** in decision-making obligatory. The patient should be provided with clear, comprehensible information about the expected benefits and risks of the procedure. In particular the patient should be made aware of the risk of death or serious complications such as stroke. In the case of the transcatheter aortic valve replacement, the patient should understand the still prevalent uncertainty about long-term benefits and risks of TAVI and valve durability (Boothroyd 2013). The intervening physician must provide information about the risks and benefits of different strategies to the patient and family and balance also the benefit of thorough discussion, perhaps requiring time for reflection, with the benefits of rapid intervention [14].

The principle of **justice** implies that patient selection criteria are as objective and transparent as possible and that access to the procedure is fair and just. It is also the physician's duty to treat the individual patient responsibly with due consideration of other patients and stakeholders in the health care system [14]. Respecting the principle of justice also requires the consideration of how decisions regarding one patient may also affect other patients and providers.

The principle of justice calls for an unbiased, equal allocation of resources that are limited. Nevertheless, "ethically speaking", medical interventions should be planned and care provided with the sole intention of improving the individual patient's quality of life and/or decreasing his or her risk of mortality "independent of reimbursement considerations and without inappropriate bias or influence from industry, administrators, referring physicians and other sources" [5].

About Ethical Problems and Issues in the Care of Geriatric Patients

An ethical problem is present when in a situation requiring a decision or an action uncertainty or disagreement arises in judging the decision or action according to the categories good and bad or right and wrong. With the aim of productively transforming this uncertainty or disagreement into a realistic course of action a process should start in which moral judgments become clear and can be expressed [31].

The response to an ethical question, the solution of an ethical problem, is not only a certain action, but in addition also an explanation and justification based on specific knowledge and facts. Thus the question by which to start an ethical case discussion should first of all aim at the course of action in the particular situation.

Here are some examples of more or less general question with ethical implications arising in everyday medical, nursing or rehabilitative care of geriatric patients. A practical suggestion how to approach them in a structured, systematic way will follow:

- What are our therapeutic, rehabilitative, nursing efforts good for? How do they make sense?
- Who is being taken care of in reality? Is it always the patient? Could it in some cases not be the patient but rather the relatives, the institution, or the society?
- The patient's will is sometimes the opposite of the benefit intended for him – how to deal with this situation?
- How does one determine the will of a patient who is not (any longer) able to communicate, like in advanced dementia, in sensory impairment, in coma?
- What is the physician's obligation to do as therapeutic intervention? What not? How to go about limiting or discontinuing active treatment?
- In medical interventions it is often easier to do everything that can be done, it is more difficult to justify not doing everything that is possible, how to go about this? Is "What can be done" and "what should be done" equivalent?
- Is curative therapy justifiable even in the end-of-life situation and how invasive may it be?
- Is the patient capable of understanding his situation, the possible clinical dilemma? Can he/she make a competent choice between the possible options?

These are concrete situations a physician can be confronted with almost daily and in which a decision has to be made. This can become particularly difficult if the patient concerned is old, frail and cognitively impaired.

Other examples of concrete clinical topics of ethical decision-making:

- Intensification, or de-escalation of invasive therapy
- Transition from curative to palliative care – when is the right moment?
- Treatment of infection or other intercurrent conditions in terminally ill patients, for example in advanced stages of dementia
- Cardio-pulmonary resuscitation – in which patients not to start? How to terminate it?

- Artificial nutrition – is it to be considered as any therapy that should be terminated when it doesn't have an indication any more, when it doesn't make sense any longer? Is there a place for PEG tubes?
- Patient abuse – particularly abuse of the elderly, frail, functionally impaired, dependent, vulnerable patient. How to recognize the various forms abuse can take? How to intervene?

Decision-Making in Geriatric Medicine

In decision-making situations as they occur frequently in everyday geriatric clinical experience – for example about the reasonability of a medical intervention it may be of help to refer to the ethical principles formulated by Beauchamp and Childress [2]. Marckmann and in der Schmitten derive from them three **legitimation preconditions** for deciding a therapeutic intervention [19],

1. The patient should have more benefit than harm from the intervention
2. The patient must give informed consent
3. The intervention must comply with state-of-the-art medical standards

A therapeutic intervention (consequently also a diagnostic one) should be abstained from if only one of these three conditions is not met. Such a renouncement of therapy based on individual ethics arguments requires a reliable judgment of the uselessness – **futility** – of a medical intervention and of the patient possibly lacking capability for consent. It can be of help to distinguish between the individual benefit and general efficacy: an intervention can be theoretically efficacious but of no usefulness or benefit for the individual patient. But it is only this individual aspect that is relevant and essential in the decision for or against a particular medical intervention.

The evaluation of the efficacy of an intervention relies on evidence from clinical trials and on clinical guidelines and/or on expert consensus recommendations based on those. Finally, the individual physician's professional expertise is also of relevance.

The presence or absence of a medical indication is the key pre-condition for initiating or foregoing a therapeutic intervention. In the absence of efficacy indication is not present – this is particularly the case in patients in the terminal stages of their lives [1].

Marckmann and in der Schmitten propose two possibilities to judge the usefulness of a medical intervention [19]:

- The narrow definition would mean that an intervention is useless if it does not have a physiological effect. This implicates well-founded professional judgment.
- The broader definition considers an intervention useless when there is a low probability of success, when the expected treatment outcomes are not desirable, when the resulting quality of life would be inacceptable, when more harm than benefit can be expected. This broader definition is judgmental it should be left to the patient capable of such a judgment.

Medical futility means that it is appropriate to withhold a therapeutic procedure from patients who are at high risk of not benefiting from it or when the expected outcome would not improve the patient's quality of life. Recognizing such situations is challenging [10].

Defining medical futility is controversial though: Schneidermann proposed that physicians "should regard a treatment as futile if empirical data show that the treatment has less than a 1 in 100 chance of benefiting the patient in a qualitatively meaningful and reliable manner" [27]. But he also admits that it is very difficult to precisely estimate expected benefit – a consensus about what constitutes the threshold of a worthwhile outcome is lacking [28].

Independence and/or Autonomy of the Geriatric Patient

Independence is frequently considered as the measure by which individual freedom and autonomy can be assessed. The gradual loss of functional independence, the risk for which is associated with aging, allegedly erodes autonomy. But functional independence should rather be related to objectively measurable somatic parameters related to the patient's specific impairment and functional capacity.

Autonomy on the other hand has a more subjective dimension that manifests itself by the individual's capacity to have self-esteem, to be free in his or her decisions, to be responsible, to evolve. A higher level of functional independence helps autonomy to manifest itself, measures of rehabilitation and care support this process.

If functional independence, like in mobility or the ability to perform activities of daily life, is not attainable it is important to confirm autonomy by not allowing for a loss of self-esteem of the individual.

The goals of geriatric rehabilitative efforts are the avoidance of dependence and improvement or maintenance of functions. Another goal of rehabilitation in geriatrics is the promotion of quality of life for the remaining years.

The mere prolongation of life is not a criterion in evaluating the positive effect of a medical intervention. "Active life expectancy" meaning life in functional health is a term that informs about a different dimension of health and morbidity, about another perspective than death alone. The end of active life expectancy is not death but the loss of functional independence and autonomy. They become an important factor of the subjective and objective appreciation of quality if life. But what about autonomy at the end of life of frail, multimorbid, perhaps cognitively impaired older persons – geriatric patients? Increasingly, autonomy is not regarded as the sole determining factor in decision-making in geriatric medicine, often times it is a rather unrealistic myth [25].

The concept of autonomy integrates essentially the notion of freedom. For Kant freedom consists of two parts: first the freedom of will, and secondly the freedom to act. The latter frequently diminishes towards the end of life as loss of functional independence progresses. If personal autonomy is supposed to be such a crucial factor of quality of life, does it mean that someone in a situation that implies progressive loss of autonomy, as in advancing cognitive impairment (dementia) cannot have and experience, enjoy quality of his or her life?

Particularly towards the end of life geriatric patients may experience a double erosion of autonomy: on the one hand through cognitive impairment (dementia), on the other through loss of functional independence with consecutive institutionalization, for example in a nursing home with its rules and regulations restricting privacy, limiting the older person's will by paternalistic rules and regulations. The principle of the individual's autonomy is undermined by the institution's principle of beneficence. Atul Gawande in his remarkable reflections on aging, frailty and the last years of life notes: "*…our elderly are left with a controlled and supervised institutional existence, a medically designed answer to unfixable problems, a life designed to be safe but empty of anything they care about…*" [9]

The reality of every-day geriatrics proves that without optimal care in the form of adequate counseling, empathy, personal attendance and assistance there would be the danger of gradually slipping into a certain "autonomism", relying on autonomous decisions of people who are no more capable of them and thus risk mainly disadvantages. A further danger would be the development of an indifferent attitude that sees only the autonomous client and disregards the consequences. According to Theda Rehbock, to accept the limitation of autonomy in advanced age with its immanent progressive need for help, support and care is a pre-condition for successful aging and contradicting the basic principle of geriatric care to do the maximum possible to preserve or to regain an optimum of independence [25].

The Patient's Will

Of course, in most situations in geriatric medicine, including the presence of cognitive impairment, decision-making is dominated and determined by the patient's will.

But one has to bear in mind, that the (presumed) will of the patient is not so relevant when there is no (longer) a meaningful medical indication for the intervention in question. According to Gian Domenico Borasio, the issue of the indication for a medical procedure has to be clarified before asking about what the patient wants. This can be done by two questions:

1. Is there a reasonable treatment goal?
2. Is this goal realistically attainable?

Only if both questions are answered affirmatively can the physician proceed to an individual appraisal of the indication and estimate whether the treatment goal is in accordance with the patient's declared or presumed preferences.

Asking for the patient's presumed will is not necessary if the therapeutic intervention in question is not indicated, if there is no reasonable therapeutic goal, or if such a goal cannot realistically be attained.

It is all about providing an indication for a medical intervention. If such an indication is not present in an individual case, then the question whether a specific intervention – for example a coronary catheterization – should be performed or not is of no relevance.

It is not so much about the specific intervention potentially performed than about the question whether it has a meaningful, attainable goal and whether its benefit outweighs the potential risks. But even before that it is about the the patient's capacity – after having been duly informed by the physician – of consenting to it or not. Such situations are clear and without ambiguity if the patient has decisional capacity, if he or she is cognitively competent. It is more difficult with a patient who is multimorbid, frail, perhaps cognitively impaired, of advanced age and approaching the end of his or her life.

A Practical Approach to Ethical Decision-Making in Individual Situations

According to Erich Loewy it is all about posing the right questions, not about expecting and following fixed instruction manuals (cook book recipes) for the particular, individual situation that poses an ethical problem. The questions can be formulated in a structured, systematic way – this would make it easier to find an appropriate individual answer. Two questions should be clarified first:

1. Who is entitled to make a decision?
2. Who is it all about (who is being treated, who wants the treatment)?

To illustrate the ethical decision-making process Erich Loewy utilizes the metaphor of planning a voyage: in it the ethicist has the role of a travel agent who places three questions in a logical fixed order (Loewy 1995):

- The first question "Where does the voyage start from?" explores the present situation. This "status quo" question is primarily a medical-technical one: physicians, nurses, therapists have to inform about the diagnosis, the prognosis and about problems still to be clarified. The ethics consultant has to make certain that experts have been involved and that the patients and his or her relatives have been adequately informed. If there is disagreement in the team on clinical issues not even the best ethicist can help.
- The second question "Where does one want to go?" is the "quo vadis" question. The one that asks about the desired goal, the destination. It is not such a medical-technical one. The physician provides the prognosis, says what is the best, what the most probable scenario. Other than that this question has mostly a biographical character: the patient's values, personal history, ambitions, goals determine the answer.
- The third question "How do we arrive at the desired destination?" is about the means to attain the goal. It is a technical question like "Should we do the coronary

intervention?" which frequently is the wrong first question before one even knows where the voyage should go.

To connect these three points – facts, goal, means to arrive at it – should now be easier.

In Geriatric Medicine one frequently has to deal with patients whose decisional capacity can be questioned because of cognitive deficits. The capacity for informed consent frequently is just a gradual one and it may be sufficient for the problem at issue. From an ethical point of view it should be possible to obtain informed consent after providing adequate information adapted to the situation, to the issue to be decided about and to the cognitive capacity of the patient.

Pre-conditions for accepting a decision – even when decisional capacity is in doubt because of cognitive impairment are:

- sufficient knowledge
- sufficient time for reflection
- authenticity
- absence of external pressure or coercion – for example social pressure

There are criteria for acceptability of a decision:

- the patient has to know the facts
- he or she has to be aware of alternative options for the therapeutic interventions
- he or she has to be capable of clearly communicating his or her preferred option
- he or she has to be capable of explaining it and of declaring that it is in accordance with his or her values – regardless if the physician shares them or not.

In the absence of decisional capacity, for example in advanced cognitive impairment, it may be of help to consider the presumable will of the patient which can be elucidated in communicating wit the relatives of the patient or proxies previously designed by the patient.

This is also the function of the written patient advance directives. In the rare cases where such indications cannot be obtained it may help to reflect about what the patient certainly would not want to experience: pain, hunger and thirst, coldness, isolation… [15]

Geriatric Palliative Care

The proximity of death is a characteristic trait of geriatrics. The imperative of maintaining and prolonging life and the ethical imperative to prevent or to palliate unbearable suffering find themselves confronted. It is about actively accompanying the dying, about palliative care and finally about allowing the foreseeable, no longer avertable death.

The dying old person has to be able to count on the empathic care of the geriatrician. The duality of the curative and of the palliative paradigms of medicine can be bridged. The pre-condition for achieving this is the acceptance of the fact that after renouncing a curative goal there is much that can still be offered to the patient: when intensive, invasive interventions to prolong survival have to be relinquished, equally intensive palliative care interventions have to start to ensure good quality of life until its end.

The challenge in caring for old people at the end of their lives lies not in just keeping them neat and nourished but in providing them an opportunity to have positive experiences. The majority of people dying are of advanced age, they are geriatric patients, many of whom so far do not profit much from the recent advances of palliative care. It is never too late for palliative care though, especially in geriatrics.

At the end of life, at the latest during the dying process, forgoing life-sustaining treatment becomes necessary. The treating physician may become confronted by the demand of the patient, or relatives to actively assist him or her in dying. In such a case one has to consider that behind this demand there is the wish not to have to continue living in the present condition – palliative care's claim is to be able to ameliorate the condition perceived as unbearable by the patient. To actively assist during the dying process is a key task of palliative care. Physicians' obligations reach their ethical and (in our society) legal limits when the demand is for active euthanasia [26].

There are typical areas of tension in which geriatric medicine has to decide and to act: for example the one between the proximity of death and the obligation to secure optimal quality of life not regarding the length of the life still remaining. Another such area of conflict is the one between promoting the individual autonomy and independence on one side and securing the protection, help and care through benevolent, caring paternalism (of the institution) when the older persons are not capable of it by themselves on the other [20].

To recognize and to accept life's end and then put into this new perspective the indication for further therapeutic interventions is not always an easy task even for the experienced physician. The decision for palliative therapy and care is often delayed by obstacles for the recognition (the diagnosis) of the dying process such as:

- hopes that the patient will get better
- lack of a clear diagnosis of the condition(s) leading to death
- pursuit of unrealistic, futile interventions
- disagreement in the team in appraising the clinical situation of the patient
- not recognising or misinterpreting symptoms

To these add:

- lack of communication skills with the patient and his or her relatives
- fears not to start or to terminate a therapy
- fears to shorten life
- cultural, religious bias, legal doubts

As a consequence of this non-recognition of dying the patient and his or her relatives remain uninformed, unprepared, they receive contradicting information. The dying process is even more troubling and lacking dignity. Burdensome symptoms are insufficiently controlled, cultural, spiritual and religious needs of the patient are not met, complex difficulties in the mourning process arise for the relatives [7].

The Austrian Federal Bioethics Commission also reflected about End of Life. It issued recommendations for the terminology of medical decisions in end-of-life situations [1]. In them, death is presented as a clearly defined irrevocable state, whereas the end-of-life is described as a process ending in death, a biologically and chronologically extendible phase of life becoming even more fuzzy by applying medical interventions. The lack of a clear definition and a diagnosis for this state means that there is no exact basis for medical interventions in the end-of-life – they become a tightrope walk between prolonging life or prolonging dying, a conflict between the medically doable and the individual benefit for the patient results. In this situation classical medical patterns of decision-making based on evidence based medical facts frequently cannot be applied because such empirical facts are not available. Decision-making often is dominated by fears of failure or of legal consequences. Dying appears to be less a natural event than a medically determined and shaped process. Collision scenarios between moral conceptions of the patients and the physicians, economic constraints, medical promises and patients' expectations become imaginable [1].

The UCLA surgeon and writer Pauline W. Chen writes that therapeutic intervention at the end of life is often being taken for a synonym of hope, confusing more therapy with more love, making withdrawal from it difficult, even impossible. No to go on treating is mistaken with giving up, the physician feels more dedicated to the therapy itself than to the patient – when so much has been done already, it becomes impossible to give up all these efforts, the therapeutic fight continues until the very last hours of life meaning that healing is the only perspective [6].

In exploring issues of caring for people at the end of their lives, the ethicists Erich H Loewy and Roberta Springer Loewy developed the metaphor of "Orchestrating the End of Life" by which they emphasize the necessity of acting in an interdisciplinary team with a radical focus on the individual patient's needs that determine the melody to be played by the palliative care team [17].

The TAVI Issue – Some Ethical Considerations

Considering the invasive cardiologic intervention in the geriatric patient much discussed at the moment – the transcatheter aortic valve implantation (TAVI) – and taking into account the ethical reflections and principles mentioned above, there are some particular aspects to be noted:

One should plan and perform procedures according to standards of care and recommended guidelines, but it should be possible to deviate from them when appropriate or necessary in the care of individual patients [5]. This is particularly true for frail, multimorbid geriatric patients, as present guidelines do not yet take into account their complex situation. Therefore advice, assistance, or consultation from colleagues should be sought when such consultation would benefit the patient undergoing an invasive cardiologic intervention (Cameron 2004).

> *"And because good ethics begins with good facts, the quality of the facts themselves takes on ethical significance [16]".*

Some facts about taking care of geriatric patients with severe aortic stenosis considered for a TAVI procedure:

- There is growing evidence that geriatric measures of functional status are important outcomes and predictors of functional outcomes in elderly patients. Evidence from pooled analyses of randomized trials even suggest that comprehensive geriatric assessment of hospitalized patients may ameliorate disability and cognitive dysfunction and improve short-term survival [8].
- The importance of a multidisciplinary patient assessment by a "heart team" prior to the chosen procedure is underlined by the difficulty in assessing the age-related peri-procedural risk of elderly patients, especially in the case of a new and rapidly evolving technology, such as TAVI [32]
- Geriatricians are competent in evaluating the degree of functional deficits, of frailty and the peri-interventional risks involved, therefore they should be integrated in "heart teams" and have a substantial impact on decision-making, long-term care and rehabilitation of elderly patients with severe aortic stenosis. A frailty index calculated as summary score from geriatric assessment instruments was a strong predictor of functional decline over a 6-month follow-up period. In contrast, established risk scores of mortality among cardiac patients such as the EuroSCORE or the STS score did not predict functional decline in a Swiss study [29].
- A particularly relevant aspect of involving geriatricians in the multidisciplinary approach of the heart teams to the selection of treatment is the avoidance of expensive, high-risk, and ultimately futile procedures in patients who will have only little symptomatic benefit or improvement in quality of life. Like for example multimorbid, highly frail patients with a very limited life expectancy, irreversible left ventricular failure, severe pulmonary disease, impaired mobility as a result of neurologic or musculoskeletal disease, advanced dementia, or other systemic disease. Timely qualified palliative care should be made available for these patients [22].
- The incorporation of measures based on a comprehensive geriatric assessment (CGA) into clinical decision-making regarding the TAVI procedure is essential for providing the best possible care to this vulnerable group of patients. Implementation of CGA into clinical routine before TAVI is not only essential for decision-making, but might also help to improve prognosis of elderly patients undergoing TAVI [30].

Thus the inclusion of geriatricians in the multidisciplinary heart teams should be considered optimal clinical and ethical practice supported by clinical evidence.

There still is some concern about the quality of the evidence on which recommendations for performing the TAVI procedure are based. Norwegian authors criticize that the American and European guidelines do not provide enough evidence yet to demonstrate that the benefits outweigh the risks. According to them current evidence is not of a sufficiently high standard to justify the strong recommendation [21].

When good evidence is lacking, it may be difficult to see whether there is a conflict between the principles of **beneficence** and **non-maleficence**, it will become equally difficult to guarantee adequate informed consent which is a prerequisite for **autonomy**. The principle of **justice** means a fair allocation of resources. This requires reliable methods again based on good evidence in order to be able to compare risk and benefits of the invasive intervention for different individual patients and patient groups (Ohldieck 2014).

Thus the big ethical challenge for interventional cardiology is to provide the solid evidence of an overall benefit of the invasive procedure translating into an individually acceptable improved quality of life of the geriatric patient. Only good facts make good ethical decision-making possible.

References

1. Austrian Bioethics Commission. Recommendations for the terminology of medical decisions in end-of-life Situations. 2011. https://www.bka.gv.at/DocView.axd?CobId=46713. Accessed 9 Jan 2015.
2. Beauchamp TL, Childress JF. Principles of biomedical ethics. New York: Oxford University Press; 2001.
3. Boothroyd LJ, et al. Transcatheter aortic valve implantation: recommendations for practice based on a multidisciplinary review including cost-effectiveness and ethical and organizational issues. Can J Cardiol. 2013;6:718–26.
4. Borasio GD. Lecture at the 66th annual German Jurist's conference, Stuttgart, 20 Sept 2006.
5. Cameron AA, et al. Ethical issues for invasive cardiologists: society for cardiovascular angiography and interventions. Catheter Cardiovasc Interv. 2004;61:157–62.
6. Chen PW. Final exam – a surgeon's reflections on mortality. New York: Knopf, Random House; 2007.
7. Ellershaw J, Ward C. Care of the dying patient: the last hours or days of life. BMJ. 2003;326:30–4.
8. Ellis G, et al. Comprehensive geriatric assessment for older hospital patients. Br Med Bull. 2004;71:45–59.
9. Gawande A. Being mortal – illness, medicine and what matters in the end. Metropolitan Books, Henry Holt & Co. New York
10. Hawkins BM, et al. High-risk percutaneous coronary intervention in the Era of public reporting – clinical and ethical considerations in the care of the elderly patient with critical left main disease and shock. Circulation. 2014;129:258–65.
11. Junod JP, Martin E. Ein kurzes Lehrbuch der Geriatrie. Bern: Huber; 1984.
12. Körtner U. Grundkurs Pflegeethik. Wien: Facultas; 2004.
13. Kunzmann P. dtv Atlas der Philosophie. Munich: DTV; 1996.
14. Levine GN, et al. ACCF/AHA/SCAI guideline for percutaneous coronary intervention. Catheter Cardiovasc Interv. 2011. doi:10.1002/ccd.23438.
15. Loewy EH. Textbook of health care ethics. New York: Plenum Press; 1996.
16. Loewy EH. Ethics and evidence-based medicine: Is there a conflict? Medscape Internal Medicine. 2007. http://www.medscape.com/viewarticle/559977_2. Accessed 7 Jan 2015.

17. Loewy EH, Loewy RS. The ethics of terminal illness: orchestrating the end of life. Dordrecht: Kluwer Academic Publishers; 2000.
18. Loewy EH, Loewy-Springer R. Textbook of healthcare ethics. 2nd ed. Dordrecht: Kluwer Academic Publishers; 2004.
19. Marckmann G, in der Schmitten J. Begrenzung lebenserhaltender Maßnahmen – eine Handreichung für die Praxis auf der Grundlage der aktuellen Gesetzgebung. Dtsch Med Wochenschr. 2010;145:570–4.
20. Morrison RS, Meier DE. Geriatric palliative care. New York: Oxford University Press; 2003.
21. Ohldieck AE, et al. Implementation of transcatheter aortic valve insertion (TAVI) in clinical practice: an ethical analysis. Clin Ethics. 2014;9(2–3):96–103.
22. Otto CM, et al. Aortic-valve stenosis – from patients at risk to severe valve obstruction. N Engl J Med. 2014;371:744–56.
23. Pauer-Studer H. Einführung in die Ethik. Wien: Facultas; 2003.
24. Pöltner G. Grundkurs Medizin-Ethik. Facultas, Wien; 2002.
25. Rehbock T. Autonomie, Fürsorge, Paternalismus – zur Kritik medizin-ethischer Grundbegriffe. Z Ethik Med. 2002;3:131–50.
26. SAMW (Schweizerische Akademie der Medizinischen Wissenschaften). Medizin-ethische Richtlinien Betreuung von Patientinnen und Patienten am Lebensende. (2004, update 2012) http://www.samw.ch/de/Ethik/Richtlinien/Aktuell-gueltige-Richtlinien.html. Aaccessed 15 Jan 2015.
27. Schneiderman LJ, et al. Medical futility: its meaning and ethical implications. Ann Intern Med. 1990;112:949–54.
28. Schneiderman LJ, et al. Medical futility: response to critiques. Ann Intern Med. 1996; 125:669–74.
29. Schoenenberger AW, et al. Predictors of functional decline in elderly patients undergoing transcatheter aortic valve implantation (TAVI). Eur Heart J. 2013;34(9):684–92.
30. Schoenenberger AW, et al. Comprehensive geriatric assessment in patients undergoing transcatheter aortic valve implantation-rationale and design of the European CGA-TAVI registry. Eur Geriatr Med. 2014;5:8–13.
31. Steinkamp N, Gordinj B. Ethik in Klinik – Ein Arbeitsbuch. Neuwied: Luchterhand; 2003.
32. Ungar A. A call to action – geriatrician's experience in treatment of aortic stenosis and involvement on transcatheter aortic valve implantation. Eur Geriatr Med. 2013;4:176–82.

Index

H. Rittger (ed.), *Interventional Cardiology in the Elderly*,
DOI 10.1007/978-3-319-21142-8

O

P

Q

R

S

T

MIX
Papier aus verantwortungsvollen Quellen
Paper from responsible sources
FSC® C105338

If you have any concerns about our products,
you can contact us on
ProductSafety@springernature.com

In case Publisher is established outside the EU,
the EU authorized representative is:
Springer Nature Customer Service Center GmbH
Europaplatz 3, 69115 Heidelberg, Germany

Printed by Libri Plureos GmbH
in Hamburg, Germany